LIFE AFTER Chemotherapy

MARCELLA POWELL, TARA KAMM,
EMILY HARDIN, TINA PISER

This book was written by women whose lives have been impacted by breast cancer. All the stories you read are true. We hope that these stories reflect courage, strength, and resilience. May you care deeper, love stronger, and hug tighter. According to current statistics, 1 in 8 women in the United States will develop breast cancer at some point in their lifetime.

ACKNOWLEDGMENTS

We would like to take a moment to express our sincere gratitude to every individual who has made a lasting impact on our lives. To all the facilities, doctors, nurses, trauma teams, ICU staff, caregivers, and volunteers who have demonstrated kindness and support during our challenging times, we are profoundly thankful.

Our heartfelt thanks go to Woodlands Medical Specialty Center in Pensacola, Florida; Baptist Health Care; HCA Medical Center; Redlands Community Hospital and Ascension Medical Center for their exceptional care.

We also extend our sincere appreciation to our families, who dedicated their time to walking alongside us through these difficult circumstances, and to our children & spouses, who encouraged us to persevere.

Most importantly, we thank God for granting us the strength to endure and continue to thrive. Together, we will remain unyielding in the face of adversity.

MARCELLA'S STORY

CHAPTER 1

Receiving a cancer diagnosis was one of the final things I could ever have imagined happening to me. Even as I navigated through the myriads of challenges and adversities life had thrown my way, the thought of receiving a diagnosis of cancer seemed as distant and unreal as a far-off dream. Throughout my life, I have heard countless stories of individuals receiving cancer diagnoses, each tale filled with descriptions of battles fought and resilience tested. I had seen countless commercials promoting cancer research, featuring heartfelt narratives urging viewers to support those undergoing treatment, often accompanied by uplifting messages of hope and perseverance. Yet, despite all these experiences and observations permeating my life, I never once felt within the depths of my being that I would face such heartbreak and despair.

In stark contrast, my existence had already included profound loss and sorrow. I had grappled with the devastating heartache of losing both of my parents before I even turned twenty-seven. Their absence created a chasm in my life, a void that echoed with memories and unfulfilled aspirations. These bruising experiences etched an indelible mark on my spirit, weaving a complex tapestry of pain that formed the fabric of my understanding of human suffering. Alongside these harrowing trials was the reality of growing up in poverty, a struggle that shaped my worldview and instilled in me a gritty determination to carve out a better life, despite the odds stacked against me.

As I continued onward, I believed that I had endured my fair share of struggles. I held on to the notion that I had not only faced the most excruciating hurts life had to offer but had also emerged with resilience and strength. I had cultivated a deep understanding of the nuances of pain and sorrow, the way they could infiltrate the very essence of life, leaving scars that could either anchor us to the past or propel us toward growth. I convinced myself that I had a pain-free future ahead of me, a life where the shadows of my past would gradually recede and allow space for joy, peace, and fulfillment. I thought that through sheer force of will and a desire to embrace a brighter tomorrow, I could forge a path free from the complications and heartaches that had long defined my journey.

But life, with its startling unpredictability and inscrutable nature, had other plans for me. In an unfathomable twist of fate, I found myself standing on the precipice of a new, unanticipated battle — one that would challenge me in ways I could never have envisaged. The diagnosis came with an air of finality, a sharp and disorienting reality that cut through the veil of normalcy I had fought so hard to maintain. It felt as though a dark cloud had descended upon my life, casting a long shadow over the aspirations and dreams I had nurtured over the years.

In that moment, the world around me shifted. The mosaic of my existence, painstakingly crafted over the years, felt as though it was crumbling beneath my feet. I began to grapple with the enormity of what lay ahead, processing a complex blend of feelings ranging from fear and vulnerability to anger and an underlying resolve. The realization that I was about to embark on a battle with cancer brought forth a torrent of emotions; all the fights I thought I had already faced now felt insignificant in comparison to this new, daunting adversary.

I asked myself questions that pierced straight to my core. How could this happen to me? Wasn't I entitled to a reprieve from suffering? As I wrestled with these queries, I found myself in a deep state of contemplation, oscillating between despair and determination. What would this new journey entail? How would I navigate the uncertainty and the unknowns of treatment and recovery? Would I emerge on the other side, forever altered by this ordeal, or would I find a way to integrate this experience into my life story, allowing it to shape me without completely defining me?

The contrast between the life I had envisioned and the stark reality ahead loomed large, and I began to slowly realize that I would need to confront this challenge not only with physical fortitude but also with a deep emotional and spiritual resilience that I had cultivated through my previous experiences. It would not be easy, and the scars of my past would continue to shape my approach to this new chapter, but I knew that I had to get the strength to face the unknown once more. In that daunting moment of realization, I understood that my journey was unfolding in a way I had never anticipated — one that would require me to adapt, to grow, and to redefine what it meant to live through pain and ultimately emerge with a renewed sense of purpose and hope.

Life, in its unpredictable and often cruel manner, chose to inflict pain upon me yet again. It felt as though I was caught in an unending cycle of anguish, where it seemed that each time I began to find my footing, life would sweep the rug out from under me. At this point in my journey, I was utterly baffled and disoriented. I grappled with the absurdity of it all — this was not a lottery system, nor was it a game of chance from which a few would come out unscathed. It was a stark and grim reality that struck without warning, reminding me of the fragility of existence.

The harsh truth settled in my mind: even the healthiest people, those who are living vibrant and full lives, can be blindsided by cancer. Disease, in all its terrifying forms, does not discriminate; it does not care about race or religion, societal status, or personal choices. I had long accepted this fact, yet it did little to temper the sense of injustice that surged within me. I was dedicated to my health, my fitness, and my spirituality, and the idea that something as ruthless as cancer could invade the sanctity of my life felt like a betrayal on a cosmic level.

In my case, I had taken measures to determine my genetic predisposition. I underwent testing for the BRCA1 and BRCA2 gene mutations, both of which came back negative. This knowledge was supposed to offer me a semblance of peace, but it did nothing to prepare me for the moment when the doctor spoke those devastating words: "You have Cancer." The weight of those words crashed over me like a tidal wave.

I vividly remember the doctor's voice continuing to speak, outlining treatment options and potential outcomes, but the words became a blur, lost in the cacophony of emotion swirling within me. My heart raced as my mind raced even faster, grappling with a multitude of questions: How could this be happening? Why was my body betraying me in such a significant way? Wasn't I supposed to be safe from this kind of suffering? I felt an acute sense of vulnerability, surrounded by a sea of uncertainty, unsure of what ahead.

In the days that followed, I found myself caught in a whirlwind of thoughts and feelings, awash with fear, sadness, and a desperate need to regain some semblance of control over my life. Friends and family rallied around me, offering their support and love, but even their well-intentioned words could not fully grasp the depth of what I was experiencing. I felt like I was on an isolated island, surrounded by a vast ocean of despair, unable to convey the magnitude of my internal struggle.

There was a constant battle between hope and despair, each vying for dominance over my psyche. I grappled with the looming unknowns of treatment, survival, and the potential long-term impacts on my life. I tried to cling to hope, searching for it in the faces of my loved ones, but it often felt like a fragile flicker against the overwhelming darkness that threatened to engulf me.

CHAPTER 2

My journey became not just one of battling a physical illness but of navigating the intricate labyrinth of emotional and spiritual upheaval that accompanied such a diagnosis. I began to realize that I was called not only to confront the realities of cancer but also to acknowledge the profoundly transformative power of fear, resilience, and faith in the face of the unknown. Life had indeed chosen me, but in that choice, there was an invitation to discover a deeper strength and purpose than I ever thought was possible.

Even before I underwent the biopsy that would confirm my worst fears, I could feel something was deeply amiss within my body. It was as if my body had begun to send up warning flares, signals that only I could interpret. Some people have remarked on how attuned I am to my own physical state, suggesting that my heightened awareness may stem from a deep connection I possess with my body. Others have proposed that it is due to the abiding presence of the Holy Spirit within me, guiding my intuition and granting me insight into my condition long before the medical community could provide clarity.

Now, as I sit here at the age of thirty-four, I find myself reflecting upon that pivotal day when I was diagnosed with breast cancer at the tender age of thirty-one. As I attempt to make sense of the journey that began on that pivotal day, I am constantly reminded that the process of grappling with a cancer diagnosis is as much an emotional and spiritual journey as it is a physical one. The ever-present sensation that something was wrong within me, coupled with the realization that my life had irreversibly changed, propelled me into an exploration of my faith, my health, and the resilience of the human spirit. It also prompted an introspection about my connection to my body and the divine, one that continues to guide me in navigating the uncharted waters of healing, hope, and redemption.

During that particular time in my life, I found myself in what I would consider to be the pinnacle of health and wellness that I had ever experienced. I was dedicated to living a lifestyle that revolved around fitness, working out consistently four to five times each week, and as a result, I had lost over eighty pounds. This incredible transformation was not merely physical; it was accompanied by a profound spiritual awakening. I had fully committed my life to God, striving to embrace and live according to His word in every aspect of my daily existence. I felt a sense of purpose, and the bonds I formed through my faith added a dimension of fulfillment that I had never before known.

Despite this newfound health and spiritual commitment, I found myself grappling with a harrowing question that shook the very foundation of my faith. It was unfathomable to me that, out of all the heinous acts of violence and atrocities occurring in the world — the murders, the rapes, the pure evil that humans inflict upon one another — God would allow such a devastating and painful experience to befall me, His beloved child. In those dark moments, I felt utterly abandoned by God, as if the connection we once shared had been severed, leaving me stranded in a state of confusion and despair.

This feeling of betrayal spiraled into a crisis of faith, leading me to contemplate if perhaps I was being punished for actions in my past. My mind raced with questions and doubts, and I found myself deeply introspective about my life choices. I began to plead my case to God, articulating a heartfelt discourse about my journey and the good I had strived to contribute to my community. I reminded Him of the countless hours I had dedicated to community service, the mentoring sessions I'd conducted, and the ways in which I had worked to uplift others, even when my own childhood was fraught with difficulties and challenges that could have led me down a far darker path.

I was determined to convince God that I had, despite my not-so-ideal beginnings, managed to turn my life around and had achieved a measure of success that I felt was commendable. It left me stunned and grappling to understand why I was now faced with the formidable diagnosis of cancer. Darkness loomed over me, and I couldn't help but ask, "Why me? Why cancer?" I felt unprepared to accept that this cruel twist of fate could befall someone who had worked so hard to better themselves and to live a life steeped in goodness and faith.

The diagnosis was not just a form of suffering; it felt as though I had been unjustly sentenced, akin to a judge imposing a twenty-year prison term for a crime I had not committed. The weight of this perceived unfairness bore down on me with relentless pressure, leaving me reeling. I was engulfed in a turbulent torrent of emotions — anger, confusion, despair — all intertwining with my longing for understanding and reconciliation with God. Each day became a battle where I wrestled not just with the physical ramifications of my condition, but with the deep, existential questions that arose within the throes of my anguish.

How could this be part of a divine plan? How could a loving God allow such suffering to enter the lives of those who were striving to follow Him? Each prayer became an outpouring of my heart, a desperate attempt to bridge the chasm I felt had opened between us. I was yearning for answers, for some semblance of clarity amidst the chaos of my emotions — a glimmer of hope or a whisper of reassurance that I was not forgotten or forsaken in my time of need.

During a particularly challenging six-month period of my life, I found myself engulfed in a whirlwind of intense emotional distress, which manifested in a seemingly constant stream of tears that marked the flow of my days. Each morning, I would wake to the oppressive weight of my feelings, and as I went about my day, tears often would slip silently down my cheeks, uninvited yet ever-present — a testament to the turbulence that existed beneath the surface of my otherwise ordinary life.

Amid this emotional turmoil, I stumbled upon a refuge, a bastion of solace that was surprisingly mundane yet extraordinarily comforting — the shower. As the warm water cascaded over my body, I allowed myself to release the pent-up sorrow that had taken residence in my heart. In that intimate space, enveloped by steam and the rhythm of water, I found a sacred sanctuary where the tears could flow freely, merging with the stream of the shower, washing away not only the evidence of my grief but, in some small part, the grief itself. This ritual became both an embodiment and a reflection of my shattered state of mind, a silent testament to the chaos and confusion that reigned within me.

Amidst the emotional upheaval, I gleaned a significant realization: during such times of tumultuous feeling and disarray, achieving clarity can feel haphazard or even impossible. I vividly recall the metaphor that echoed in my mind, one that illustrated my predicament beautifully: the experience of dropping a pair of glasses. When the lenses become crooked or misaligned, the world viewed through them is a distorted tapestry of shapes and colors, rendering the reality around you unclear and hard to grasp. It is only when the lenses are returned to a professional — such as the manufacturer or an optician — that they can be adjusted and restored to their proper function, allowing the wearer to regain true vision and see the world with clarity once more.

Similarly, I came to understand that I was in a metaphorical fog, obscured and unable to see the bigger picture or the purpose behind the pain I was experiencing. It wasn't until I opened my heart and mind to the possibility of divine intervention that I began to sense a new direction emerging from my despair. This process of seeking a relationship with God — engaging with my spirituality and drawing upon the strength and understanding found in faith — allowed me to peel back the layers of confusion and start delving deeper into my life's circumstances.

As I engaged in this introspective journey, I began to uncover insights that transcended my immediate suffering. I realized that my struggles held meaning and that they were not without purpose. This newfound purpose began to illuminate my path through the darkness, like light breaking through a thick fog. I understood that the emotional distress I faced was not just a random act of fate or a simply unfortunate phase of my life; instead, it reflected a deeper narrative that was urging me toward growth and understanding.

Thus, through this period of persistent trials and tribulations, I found myself on a transformative journey, learning the valuable lesson that even in our most profound sorrows, there lies the potential for insight and clarity, as well as the opportunity for personal evolution. The key, I have come to understand, is to embrace the pain and seek out the lessons hidden within it, leading to a path that, though initially obscured, may ultimately reveal a profound sense of purpose and resolution.

CHAPTER 3

As I navigate through my current journey of recovery, I have come to firmly believe that life after experiencing cancer is not merely an existence defined by an ailment or a disease but rather an embodiment of what life truly is in its essence. The truth, as I see it, is that the former way in which I lived my life has irrevocably concluded, and the individual I once identified as has essentially faded away. The old version of me is not the same person standing here today. This transformation has been profound, fundamentally altering my mindset and reshaping my actions in ways that I never could have envisioned prior to this experience.

In essence, I hold the conviction that life after cancer is simply life because it has opened my eyes to a more profound comprehension of what it truly means to exist and to thrive. This newfound understanding is rooted in the recognition of the preciousness of every moment. Before my diagnosis, I was often tethered by fear — fear of taking risks in various aspects of my life, whether that be in pursuing new business opportunities, engaging with new people socially, or making the difficult but necessary decision to let go of relationships that no longer served me well. The challenge posed by cancer imparted an invaluable lesson: tomorrow is never promised, and with this realization comes the core understanding that we must embrace the strength and vitality we experience today, even though the possibility of immense pain may loom on the horizon.

Reflecting on this reality, I have found myself pondering a series of questions. Why refrain from taking a chance on something that could change my life for the better? Encouraged by this thought, I took the leap. Why not permit myself to let go of all that weighs me down and prevents me from moving forward? In a moment of clarity and courage, I chose to release the burdens I had carried for far too long. Why not embark on new journeys and experiences that could enrich my life? With a heart full of hope and determination, I took that first step into the unknown.

Within the chaos and challenges of the past, I discovered a surprising and beautiful resilience that emerged from what initially felt like a disastrous situation. This process has profoundly impacted my perspective, leaving me with a deep and abiding sense of gratitude for life itself. I have learned to appreciate the small moments — the fleeting experiences that many may overlook in their daily hustle. I have come to realize that life is not merely a chronology of days divided by significant milestones; rather, it is about the richness of the moments we create and the connections we foster.

In embracing this new outlook, I find joy in the simple and the profound — whether it's the laughter shared with friends, the warmth of the sun on my face, or the peacefulness of a quiet evening spent in reflection. Each of these elements contributes to my evolving understanding of existence post-cancer: every single day is an opportunity waiting to be seized, and I am determined to live each one fully and authentically. This journey has been life-changing, sparking not only a shift in how I perceive my own existence but also a deep appreciation for the beauty and complexity of life itself in all its forms.

Navigating the myriad of obstacles, I encounter, both in terms of my physical well-being and the occasional toll on my mental state, proves to be an arduous journey, yet I am constantly reminded that life continues to unfold around me. My diagnosis forced me into a crossroads, one in which I had to make some of the most significant decisions regarding my health and treatment. After considerable contemplation and following deep discussions with my oncologist, I concluded that undergoing chemotherapy presented the most promising opportunity to minimize the risk of cancer returning in the future.

However, embracing that path was not without its consequences. I had to firmly acknowledge that the chemotherapy treatment, while potentially lifesaving, came together with a host of side effects that I now must endure on a daily basis. Upon choosing to proceed with the chemotherapy regimen, I was inundated with an overwhelming amount of information that spanned across ten pages of printed material. Strikingly, eight of those pages were filled with densely packed text in minuscule print, which served as disclaimers, aiming to provide a comprehensive overview of what this treatment entailed, and the possible ramifications associated with it. These pages were intended to cover crucial information, yet for someone already grappling with the emotional strain of a cancer diagnosis, being requested to absorb so much information was a monumental task.

The sheer volume of details and the complex medical jargon only intensified the mental overload I was experiencing. I was wrestling with a swirl of emotions — fear, apprehension, and confusion — as my mind grappled with the harsh reality of my situation. Confronted with the weight of my diagnosis, the gravity of the treatment decision loomed large, and the uncertainty of what lay ahead was nothing short of paralyzing. It felt as if my thoughts were being drowned out by the chorus of voices echoing in my mind — well-meaning friends and family, medical professionals offering advice, and my own anxiety. Each voice clamored for attention, creating a cacophony that made it increasingly difficult for me to find clarity amid the chaos.

Amidst this tumult, I realized that one of the most significant challenges I faced was understanding how to find stillness in my heart and mind, allowing me to foster a deeper connection with God to hear His guidance amidst the clamor of concerns and distractions. This journey represents a delicate balancing act, navigating through the fog of uncertainty while striving to cultivate a spirit of peace and faith. Although finding that quiet space within me was challenging, I hold onto the belief that achieving this connection is not only possible but essential for my sense of well-being. With each day that passes, I remain determined to silence the noise in my head, creating an inner sanctuary where I can truly listen and reflect on my faith, allowing it to guide me through this daunting path ahead.

Agreeing to undergo chemotherapy, a decision I made without fully grasping the extensive implications that would accompany the treatment, has dramatically altered not only my physical health but also my overall quality of life in ways I could never have anticipated. The reality of living with the consequences of this choice has unfolded itself in a particularly harsh manner; from the moment I rise in the morning to greet the day until I finally ease into sleep at night, the experience of genuine comfort has become an elusive notion, rarely gracing me with its presence.

This unending struggle with discomfort has thrust me into a precarious position where I must confront a formidable decision: should I allow myself to be overwhelmed by this adversity, accepting defeat as my fate, or should I muster every ounce of strength within me to resist and strive for victory, however that may be defined? Although my body may be operating beneath its optimal levels and frequently feels like it is in an uphill battle against itself, I adamantly refuse to see defeat as a viable option.

Since embarking on this journey through chemotherapy, I have been led to interact with a multitude of medical professionals. My struggles range widely, including issues such as hormonal imbalances, chronic dizziness, autoimmune disorders, persistent chronic pain, neuropathic symptoms, and a plethora of dental complications. Yet, this catalogue of physical difficulties does not begin to scratch the surface of my daily reality. There are numerous symptoms that I contend with that have yet to be adequately addressed by any healthcare provider, including but not limited to memory loss, slurred speech, profound exhaustion, deep bone aches, various skin rashes, psychological trauma, and pervasive feelings of depression and anxiety.

It is particularly noteworthy that anxiety stands out as the only symptom in this extensive list that I did experience prior to starting chemotherapy. The arrival of anxiety has added another layer of complexity to my already challenging existence, leaving me to navigate this unfamiliar emotional terrain while simultaneously managing the physical ramifications of my treatment. The overall experience has been a complex interplay of battling both the physical and mental health effects that have emerged as a direct result of my decision to pursue chemotherapy. In this ongoing battle, I continue seeking ways to reclaim my sense of normalcy amid the chaos, striving to carve out moments of peace and resilience against the waves of adversity that my journey has brought.

— Marcella Powell

TARA'S STORY

CHAPTER 4

I remember when I was first diagnosed, I went through this weird thought pattern where I actually wanted to do chemo. Because if I needed to do chemo, then this cancer diagnosis was "real." Somehow, in my mind, the battle would not seem as "real" or "significant" if I didn't have to do chemo. How twisted is that? As if cancer wasn't really cancer if you don't have to fight for your life?!

These are the weird things that your brain does when you hear the word cancer. The intrusive thoughts crept in almost immediately into the journey for me. I'd ask myself, "What is wrong with me? Why am I thinking like this? Do I actually want it to be cancer? Do I actually want to do chemo and radiation?" "Why would I want to have to do these treatments?" Personally, I think it's a safety net we create for ourselves, so we don't fall too far mentally. Like, if I allowed myself to have the intrusive thoughts and allowed myself to assume the worst, then I could navigate the actual battle better.

What if I told you that I'm not the only one who has these thoughts? That this is a completely normal way to process things? We need to allow ourselves the headspace to work it all out. Unfortunately, what I did was allow myself to jump off a mental cliff! I went deep and dark fast! And the truth is I never needed to! When the diagnosis was survivable, I had to mentally figure out a way to climb back up the cliff and out of the dark pit of death and dying! Which was a hard climb back up. You must climb back up, though, because positivity and outlook are the number one way to beat this diagnosis! And I wanted to live! The first battle is in the mind.

Cancer ended up being more than just a health issue; it brought to light wounds I've carried for years and never dealt with. Things I repressed deep within myself. Funny how it all comes to the surface when life is, in fact, threatened. You realize how short life can be and what a gift it is while you are here! Then you have to decide what kind of life you want to live and ask, am I doing it? If not, it's time to start living that life now! That is exactly my goal now. But before I can tell you about life after chemo, I need to give you some of my journey.

How It Began, Again

The way back… I found a lump in my breast when I was around 32 years old. Imaging showed it to be an atypical cyst, and it required monitoring for five years. But, on the fifth year of monitoring, my husband changed jobs and we lost our insurance for a few months. Once the insurance got squared away, I hesitated to go in for the final imaging. So, I was almost a full year late for the last image. Now, I know that it was all in God's timing! If I had gone in when I was scheduled to go, it would have been clear, and I would have been released until I was 40. So, the delay kept me from having cancer then. It was pre-cancerous calcifications that I had to have surgically removed with a lumpectomy. They suggested I go see an oncologist, and I ignored the suggestion out of fear. In hindsight, I sure wish I had not ignored the fact that my body was sending me warning signals!

Fast forward to the worst year ever: 2020! I am now 41 years old. I had faithfully gone every year for my mammogram. It had been clear for six years. Then the year from hell.

At the time, I was seeing a local doctor who was more holistic in her approach to medicine. I have been very healthy since having my children. I am organic, non-GMO, and moderately healthy in my food choices. I try to live by the thought that if God didn't make it, then I shouldn't eat it. Also, with that being said, I will eat the cake if it's there and have some wine occasionally. I was by no means the picture of health, but for the most part, I was much better than most in this department. After a ruptured appendix in 2019, I was desperately trying to rebuild my health. The massive rounds of antibiotics given to save my life damn near killed me! So, I was trying to rebuild my gut health and seeing this very expensive holistic doctor. I just didn't feel good. I couldn't say what I thought it was or what direction to go. I just knew something was wrong, and I just didn't feel like myself.

Is it really this downhill at 40? That is what everybody always says! After much blood work and testing, the doctor found my white blood cell count was high and she thought I may have a hidden infection in my body and planned to do some crazy test to trace the white blood cells to find the infection. Her decision was due to the peritonitis I had after the ruptured appendix. She was thinking maybe the antibiotics didn't get all the infection out. This test she ordered was not covered by insurance and, oh, by the way, it costs upwards of $5,000! I said fine, but before we do all that, I am due to get my mammogram. Then it all began. Again.

The day I got the call for needing more diagnostic imaging, I was having a hard day in a big way. So, when I hung up with the nurse, I cried. Hard. This was a weird reaction to the call, but I chalked it up to the stressful time I was in. I've known this nurse for years through my journey at this facility. She said, "The calcifications are back, and we need to see a place on the right side as well." In my gut, I just knew it was cancer. But maybe it was just stress...maybe.

We were in the middle of a global pandemic from COVID; my job had been shut down for a few months, and I was unable to get government help. A hurricane had come a few months prior and flooded under our home. We lost a car, belongings, and our septic tank! So, I was dealing with insurance claims. The hurricane took out the main bridge in our town and caused a major disruption to life for an entire year! Also, a lawsuit I had been a part of for several years was finally moving forward in the worst way. When I say it was a stressful time, I mean so, so, so stressful!

All in all, I felt I was handling it all okay. Until the call. I cried and let it all out. All the emotions I had been suppressing through this season of hard! After I cried, I told myself I was ridiculous for being so fearful and emotional! Why do I always make everything such a big deal? I scheduled the follow-up imaging for a day I would be in town; due to the bridge being out, I wanted to squeeze it all in when possible. I would go to work, see one patient, then run to get the imaging, and then back to work. I am a dental hygienist and thankfully work for the best office, and they allowed me to have this flexibility.

When I got to the imaging center, I asked to speak to the radiologist before leaving that day. They said it was no problem. I had already gotten the mammogram, and they took me in for an ultrasound. I'm not sure if they were out of gowns or if this was routine. They gave me a washcloth-sized towel to cover myself with while getting the ultrasound. In the middle of the imaging, a man walks in while I am lying down, essentially exposed. He says, "You wanted to talk to me; I am the radiologist." I said, "Yes, I wanted to talk to you, but not like this!" He ignored the fact that I was lying down, basically exposed, and covering myself with my hands. So, I said, "I just wanted to hear from your mouth that I am okay; the calcifications are back, and I want to hear from you that it's nothing." He says, "Oh, yeah, it's nothing to worry about; just some residual calcifications from your previous biopsy." He turns and leaves the room, and the tech follows him.

So, I assume we are done, and I get up to get dressed, all while feeling like I want to throw up. I felt physically nauseous. I figured it must be because he was so abrupt and abrasive. And I felt exposed. God has given me the gift of discernment, and I can usually read and decide if I like someone within seconds. So, that must be why I feel so sick. I just didn't like him or the situation! He came back in the room, followed by the tech and looks annoyed that I am up and dressed. He says, "We aren't done; she needs to show me something." I say, "Well, I already got dressed." He says, "It's fine; just lift your shirt." I've never even lifted my shirt at Mardi Gras and yet somehow, I would have felt more comfortable there! He is pretty adamant, so I lift my shirt. The tech points to the screen and says, "Here is the spot we've been watching...but what is that?" He barely even looks at the screen and says, "It's nothing; she is fine."

I say, "While you are in here, let me ask again. You say it's residual from my biopsy, but I had surgery! There has not been any residual for six years and now the calcifications are back. Are you SURE I'm fine?" He looks at me harshly, lifts his hand to dismiss me, and says, "Yeah, how old are you?" I said, "41." He said, "Yeah, you're fine. I'll go get your paperwork to release you for the year." All the while I am so nauseous. So, I decide to pray. I asked God, "Why do I feel this way? What am I feeling? Is it him I don't like or is it something else?" Then, instantly, I start praying, "God, if it's something, make him see it! Make him see it...make him see it..." on repeat in my mind.

All while fighting more thoughts of "What is wrong with me? Do I want it to be something? Do you want it to be cancer? Are you crazy? Just be happy he's releasing you and you got good news! Why are you so dramatic?... God, please make him see it!" He returns to the room and has my release paperwork already signed. I sign it too, and I can't help but ask again. "So, again I ask you. I had surgery and have had no residual calcifications all this time, and you are positive it is nothing to worry about." He says, "Yeah, you are fine. See you next year." He leaves the room. I keep praying! Me and the tech joke about how "great he is" and how "he must be so fun to work with." She laughs and states he is pretty awful and always like this! All the while, I am still praying! "God, make him see it..." She started to escort me out of the double doors to leave when I hear someone running behind me. I turned around to see what was happening. I've seen enough movies to know I may need to run or get out of the way! What I see instead is the radiologist running toward me, saying, "WAIT...Don't leave... it's complicated!"

This is how I began my breast cancer journey. And every step of the journey was just as hard and just as bad as this! So, why share this? To get you angry for me? To make you fearful? No, not at all. I share this for two reasons.

Number One: Never underestimate the power of prayer! I received answered prayer! God made that man go back and actually look through my records and imaging. Then this man swallowed his pride and ran after me to stop me. He admitted his wrong, and this saved me a year of metastasis. Later, I found out that the cancer was already in my lymph nodes and grade three, which is the most aggressive and likely to metastasize. This man could have ignored God and let me leave. But God said NO! Not today! Thank you, Jesus! I am so very thankful that instead of focusing on my thoughts, fears, and emotions that I decided to pray! How often do I get that right? Prior to this moment, not often, but after this moment, I get it right most of the time! Now I know when I feel this strongly, I need to pray! I need to put my thoughts aside and ask God what He is trying to tell me or show me! I will never ever ignore that feeling again! Prayer is the answer every single time!

Number Two: How often do we as women quiet that voice inside that tells us to push? Tells us to ask the question three times? The voice that says, "This is not right!" So often, we keep quiet when we are called to speak! We have heard throughout history how dramatic women are and how difficult women can be! We've even thought this about other women more often than we would like to admit! But what if that voice was the prompting of the Holy Spirit? What if that "feeling" is the prompting from the Lord? When did we women decide to stay quiet? I say, from now on, when I feel led to speak, I will! I will say the hard things. I will ask the hard questions. And I will listen when something feels "off" inside of me! Now I know what that feels like, and I will never ever ignore it again! We HAVE to be our own advocates in this life! We have to start speaking when led! The intrusive thoughts I had were nothing more than the enemy trying to keep me quiet...no more! Had I not spoken up and prayed, this battle I faced would have been much harder and could have cost me my life.

CHAPTER 5

I will spare you the details of my treatment and most of the things I faced! Just know that every step of the way I was asking myself, "How can the health industry be this broken?" I was diagnosed with invasive ductal carcinoma with lobular features, stage 2, grade 3, ER+PR+HER2-. I did four rounds of chemotherapy — Taxotere and Cytoxan — followed by 33 rounds of radiation to my chest, sternum, armpit, and neck. I had no genetic factors, and no one in my family had ever had breast cancer except my grandmother on my dad's side. She got it when she was in her seventies, so they say that it isn't connected due to her age. I told the doctor that since mine was caused by my hormone imbalance, it was, in fact, genetic. Every woman on my mom's side and my dad's side had to have a full hysterectomy before the age of 40 due to major hormonal issues. Some had tumors and cancer, and some just had hormonal imbalance issues. At 41, I was the oldest woman in my family to still have her parts. So, please, someone tell me how that isn't genetic! The doctor simply stated that science is changing all the time and new research will come out for years ahead. I said, "Well, since 80% of all breast cancer is caused by a hormone imbalance, it seems that maybe research should start there!"

I digress. Because I am a dental hygienist, I have an associate of science degree and have taken all the same courses as a nurse. I am a licensed health professional. I believe that the mouth is the window to the health of the body! I love to educate my patients and help them understand this and why oral health is so important. That is just the mouth and teeth. I expected to get this kind of education on cancer! I expected the same standard of care that I give my patients. I expected to have my hand held and to be totally educated on the drugs they were using and what to expect with my body. That is not what happened. I got no chemo class. I got no education on anything! Nada, zip, zilch! I asked questions and got runaround answers! So, I started asking questions on purpose to see what they would say! The answers were simply shocking! I was amazed at how little the nurses seemed to know about chemo and its effects. I think by now we all know how the health industry is run. Most likely, insurance is pulling the strings and the doctors and nurses are overworked with minimal help. But to have no education given to me was astounding.

So far, I may sound negative towards it in general, but let me stop here and say that I am SO thankful for the doctors and nurses that saved my life and killed my cancer! They did exactly what they had to do. And so far, it worked! So, for that, I am beyond grateful! But how can the health industry be this broken? I asked why I didn't get a chemo class and was told that they don't do that anymore. But if I had any questions, they would be happy to answer them for me. How in the world would I know what to ask?

When I had a side effect from the chemo, I'd call my oncologist team and they would tell me that it could not be connected because my dose was too low. I'm sorry, what? Please, please don't diminish the fact that you are putting chemical drugs into me and I am, in fact, reacting! So, they would send me to a specialist to find the cause. The specialist would seem annoyed and tell me that it's common from my chemo! I would return from the specialist and no one would address the issues I was having. When I finally had enough from the facility I was getting treatment from, I requested my records. They printed out my paper chart and it was about three inches thick. I sat down one evening alone with a glass of wine and a highlighter. I went through every page and none of my symptoms were ever documented! NONE! When I tell you it was bad...I mean it was bad!

My body after chemo will never be the same. As a woman in her 40s, I often wonder if it's just age or if it's from the chemo/radiation. I honestly will never know. Not only did the doctors diminish the side effects of the drugs, they made it seem like life goes on as normal. They downplayed all the symptoms I had and made me feel like I had done something to bother them. I actually felt like they hated me! I am a pretty compliant person and wasn't a problem patient at all! I know I sound strong-willed and difficult, but I promise I never went in with anything but the love of God! It was important for me to show them the love I felt from God. I wanted and felt like this was a mission field. So, to receive this treatment from them was very hard to swallow! I will never know if I had any impact on them on this side of heaven, but they certainly had an impact on me! As far as health, all I can say is, what was "normal" is long gone.

After chemo, you are forever changed. It ages you on a cellular level. It changes everything. After the battlefield, you stand victorious and are called a "warrior"! But you no longer recognize the person looking back at you in the mirror! I felt like I was beat up and tossed aside. Chemo attacks everything that makes you feminine! All of it. Because my cancer was from my hormones, I opted to have a full hysterectomy. So, now I also have no essential hormones. I am experiencing menopause symptoms at rapid onset. Forced into menopause from chemo and completed with a hysterectomy. Menopause comes with a LONG list of side effects in itself! So, is it chemo or is it menopause? It's both!

The medical team and our friends and families all seem to think that you should just bounce back to "you." But honestly, the old you is dead and gone. A new you has emerged, and you never even had time to mourn the loss of your old self or become acquainted with this new person. And to be honest, I didn't like this new version one bit! She gained 20 pounds from the steroids and she is always hot, bald, sweaty, and very tired! She has aches all over her body and can't quite hang like she used to! All I can say is that it really is like you stepped off a battlefield. I imagine soldiers coming home from fighting in a war have a new version of self as well. And life just goes on for everyone around them. How do you find your footing after such a battlefield? How do you essentially start over? That was and is my mission: to find out about this new version of me, get to know her, and get her into good health. I was determined to take back what cancer stole from me! This is my mission. So, after some much-needed time to heal and recover, I started seeking God, asking, "Okay, God, what is next?" Like always, He was faithful to answer me!

CHAPTER 6

Like I said, the old me is dead and gone! Thank God for that! Yes, I am still suffering from menopause and long-term side effects of chemo… I definitely have some white coat syndrome with a touch of PTSD at doctor visits!! But aside from that, this new me is unstoppable! I have found new purpose and direction for my life! I have a new love for life and have created so many healthy boundaries in relationships! I am just getting started! I can't wait to share what God did after it was all over. And the hardest part to say out loud… I am actually thankful for cancer. I know that sounds absolutely crazy, but it is true. Let me explain.

So, I had been asking God why He was showing me all the ways the health system is broken. Why was He making me aware of how "bad" it really is? For what? What could I possibly do to change it? Somehow, I just knew He was going to use this cancer battle for His good. I felt in my soul that I can use this journey to help others. The "why" questioning went on for months! No answer. I wasn't ready yet. I had some healing to do, not just physically but emotionally and spiritually as well. I won't go into all the details here, but I had some major life obstacles and hurts that arose shortly after the cancer journey ended. Major upsets! And I thought cancer was hard! This was an entirely different battlefield, but a battle nonetheless. It made me so damn angry, and I felt like it was a righteous anger!

It wasn't until I gave it all over to God and allowed Him to help me heal from the hurts and let go of the anger that I was ready! I had to forgive. I had to forgive the doctors, the nurses, that dang radiologist, my cancer team, all the people who didn't show up when I was diagnosed, all the ones who left me high and dry, all the wounds I carried from fear, anger, and mistrust. I had to forgive them all. I wasn't ready for a while. I wanted to be mad. I deserved the right to be mad! These people had hurt me! These doctors, friends, family... it was all too much to carry. I wanted to be angry! It felt good to be angry!

Can you believe that God used my anger for good too? Maybe I had to go through these emotions in order to come out of it ready. My anger is what spurred me on. My anger is what led me to ask God all the questions. Anger is okay; it's normal to feel this way. But we can't stay angry because if we do, it starts to eat us up inside and makes us bitter and guarded. We can't very well do much for God in this state of mind now, can we? So, friend, who do you need to forgive? What wound are you carrying too? It's much too heavy, so I'd suggest laying it down at the foot of the cross and leaving it there. It will take time. There is freedom for you after forgiveness.

I will say that I do not believe that God gave me or gives anyone cancer! I believe it is an attack of the enemy to kill, steal, and destroy! He uses things like cancer and sickness to attack us. Just read the story of Job! Yes, God allowed the enemy to attack Job and to go through it all. In the end, He double blessed him for his faithfulness through the hell he walked through because Job never lost his faith! So, neither will I! If this trial is something I must face, then I will face it! The enemy only attacks those who are a threat to his kingdom! So, I must be doing something right!

Also, our diet plays a huge factor; our environment is toxic beyond belief; our stress management is poor; the chemical overload in our homes… the list goes on! Why would I believe I didn't have a role to play in my sickness as well? Why would I blame God for this? It was time to get serious about all these things. God was also showing me the realities of our environment and what role all of this plays into our sicknesses. In order to stay out of the health "industry," we need to get serious about our health.

So, the question remained: Why, God? What are you calling me to? I had healed from my anger and was walking closer to God than I had in far too long. One day, I was in my hot tub with my husband and it was a beautiful spring morning. I looked around and said how I love spring; I've always been a fall girl. But I think my season is changing. My husband laughed with me and went inside. I stayed awhile, enjoying my cup of coffee and listening to all the new baby birds chirping, seeing all the new growth on the trees, and all the flowers in bloom. The fresh smell in the air all felt like new life emerging.

I had the thought that this is the season I am in as well. I am blooming, coming out of a season of cold and harshness. A very long emotional winter, if you will. A new life emerging within me. I just felt wrapped in love in that moment. I took it all in. The next thing I know, all these thoughts just start "downloading" into my head! As the thoughts are coming in, I am agreeing with them and thinking what a good idea they are! And then I realize that God just gave me my answer! I finally knew how to use what He had shown and taught me! And it wasn't about me at all! It was amazing, and I could not wait to get started! I had so much to learn! God has a sense of humor! He called me to something I know very little about, but I was willing to learn. And I was ready!

I started a YouTube/podcast/social media channel called Power Over Pink. I am interviewing other breast cancer survivors so they can share their stories. As a woman of faith, I know just how strong our testimonies are and how important it is to share them with others. So, this direction made total sense to me. I want to share others' stories! All the stories! When we share our stories, we give ourselves a voice in a voiceless system. It helps the survivor to feel heard and seen! Not just another number being passed through a system! A life touched and forever changed from a cancer diagnosis.

When others are diagnosed and turn to the internet like I did, they will find hope and encouragement! As we listen to hear what other survivors faced, we learn what to ask, what to expect, and where to turn when we need help. Survivors have shared things like nonprofits they found that can help you along the journey, books they read, supplements they found to help, etc. In sharing our stories, we can better equip and encourage someone just entering the battlefield. I also share health tips and tricks that help along the journey and after it's over. It's never medical advice, just inspiration from women who faced it and won! In sharing, you learn how to be your own advocate and what to ask. When to speak up and push when something "feels off," and so much more! In starting the channel, I have met the most incredible women! Friendships that are so meaningful and helpful in my life! All because I was willing and ready!

This is my purpose. I love people. I love serving people, and I love sharing what God has done through it all. From cancer came life purpose and direction. I know I am just getting started, and I don't know where it will go from here. But wherever God leads, I will follow! In facing this battle, I am learning so much about myself. I have a different value of time now. I will celebrate every birthday and will tell anyone who wants to know how old I am. Because birthdays are a gift that many don't get to have. Cancer is a thief and has taken far too many lives. When we share, we also honor those lives that have been lost. In this fight, I get to show my kids how to take something terrible and make it into something amazing! This is my new life after chemo. I'm in a deeper relationship with my Father in Heaven, and He has given me a new life! I am still getting to know this new body, getting acquainted with all her new aches and pains. I have to constantly watch for those intrusive thoughts and hold them captive to the authority of Christ! Fear is a liar, and not every single pain is cancer. The difference is, after chemo, I am forever changed...for the better. What the enemy meant for evil, God certainly used for good. And I, for one, can't wait to see where this leads.

—Tara Kamm

EMILY'S STORY

CHAPTER 7

You always hear people say things like, "You never know what you have until you lose it." A bit of a cliché, but one I find most of us can agree with. These words never rang truer than when I received the news that I had breast cancer. Not only would I miss my boobs, my hair, and even my ovaries, but most of all, I'd miss the old version of myself and all of the simplistic day-to-day ruminations of ordinary life before cancer came along and set me spinning like a toy top across a marble floor.

Right before I found out, I was just your normal, average woman going about my normal, average day. I would enter the hospital nervous about receiving my test results but secure in my belief that I was perfectly healthy. Here I am, as scheduled, but let's get this over with because I must be getting on with it and back to the business of being busy!

At the time, my mind would be more concerned with the never-ending list of "mom" and work-related responsibilities that made up my routine. I had no idea that I'd leave that building in the earliest stages of a deep transformation. I would step out into the parking lot in a daze, my biopsy results clutched in my hand and tears blurring my vision, already different from who I was just that very morning while I was brushing my teeth and getting dressed. I also had no idea that everything I would lose over the next year of treatment, surgeries, and recoveries would be the catalyst for all that I would gain and learn and who I was yet to become in the aftermath of cancer.

The news felt like the ultimate betrayal. Like suddenly my body, the one that I've known my entire life, had somehow become a foreign vehicle of mystery and harm, a stranger capable of unpleasant surprises completely unbeknownst to me—the one person who was, well, living with me. This could not be the same body that carried my two children, nursed them as babies, and thus far had been relatively healthy for most of my adult life. I now had a better understanding of the term "out-of-body experience." I remember feeling as though I was no longer anchored to the seat beneath me, but that I was hovering somewhere else in the small room, a little farther to the left of myself, no longer feeling my own hands wringing nervously together in my lap as the doctor's words seemed to be coming from farther away. The doctor, whom I just met that morning, gently told me that my biopsy came back confirming that the lump was not an infected cyst as my mammogram and ultrasound initially concluded, but it was actually a cancerous tumor in my right breast.

Her eyes were so kind as she delivered this news and blew up my world. All I could do was nod as she went into the long list of next steps. I couldn't quite find my voice or conjure up any adequate questions. The word "cancer" was ricocheting around in my brain like a stray bullet. The "C" word was like a deafening bang, drowning her out. Part of me was there, listening attentively and matter-of-factly. The other part of me grappled to process the meaning of all of this. I was in complete shock and disbelief. No, she's not talking about me! I'm perfectly healthy! There's no way that I can have cancer, even if it runs in my family. I'm only 38; too young for breast cancer! I eat leafy greens occasionally and I pay my taxes! I'm a good human being! Surely not me! So rude!

It wasn't until I was sitting in the waiting area again that the enormity of the word "cancer" fully hit me. Cancer was an entomologist, and I was the insect, being pressed between the cold glass of a shadow box, squashing my safe and mundane existence along with all my big plans for the near future. I had just started a very demanding job at the time too, and the sheer inconvenience of it all was outrageous to me!

It dawned on me that suddenly, I was in the clutches of an enemy who everyone knew didn't play fair and whose rules I was unfamiliar with, and although I knew that catching cancer early enough made the odds of survival a lot higher than ever before, I couldn't help but think of every movie that I ever watched where the mom died from a long and vicious battle with cancer. I pictured myself emaciated, eyes hollow, head bald, laying in a hospital bed in my living room, with an IV hooked to my pale arm and an oxygen mask covering my wan face as my family looked on with sad eyes at the shell of what was left of me. I thought of my two kids, Rose and Raiden, 14 and 18 at the time, and how it would affect them not having a mother. That's when the tears I was holding back came trickling down, soaking the rim of the white mask that I wore in the waiting room as I struggled to blot my eyes and wipe my nose. I was hugely embarrassed to be crying in public. I looked around at the other masked strangers on the oncology floor who were very likely going through what I was soon to be going through, and I felt a mixture of guilt (some of these people probably had it much worse than me), sadness, anger, but most of all...fear.

Even though the fear of dying (What if it's late stage or terminal? What if I'm one of the ones who don't make it?) was there in the periphery, everything began to move so quickly that I immediately went into survival mode. My treatment consisted of 16 rounds of chemotherapy: 4 Adriamycin and Cytoxan, a.k.a. Red Devil, and 12 Taxol, along with a double mastectomy with immediate reconstruction, 25 rounds of radiation, a full hysterectomy due to BRCA2, and also 3 additional surgeries from complications with my left chest expander. It would be a year-long plus battle that I would emerge from much changed—physically, emotionally, and mentally.

All this said, ever the optimist, I was resolved to march into chemotherapy and blow everyone away with my great attitude and unwavering positivity. Birds would land on my outstretched fingertips and forest creatures would gather around me because I would be a wholesome beacon of quiet, unshakeable strength. I would be the self-proclaimed Disney princess of chemo—Chemorella, if you will. This vision of myself seemed entirely plausible to me. That is, until I received my first round of A.C. Adriamycin & Cytoxan, better known as the Red Devil because of its red color—and because, apparently, the thought of chemo isn't scary enough, so why not give it an intimidating nickname? My honest opinion after the first round? This shit sucks! Would not recommend the Red Devil. One star on Google Reviews.

It's important to note that everyone responds differently to chemo. My biggest side effects with A.C. were severe nausea, headaches, dry mouth, and fatigue. I once heard it compared to feeling like a full-body hangover without having had any of the fun at the party, and based on my experience, that sadly is a very good description.

For many, chemo side effects are cumulative. I received A.C. once every two weeks, and each time I took it, it took me a little longer to recover before it was time to go in for the next infusion. My hair fell out about 2 weeks after the second round, and I felt sicker, weaker, and more tired than I have ever felt before in my life. I looked in the mirror and saw a much older woman. With the loss of my hair, what I considered my femininity seemed to melt away overnight, and I was left looking at a complete stranger. It was then that it became very real that I was indeed a cancer patient.

I mourned my old life. I missed having the energy to go jogging with my dog, to dance in my house when a good song came on the radio, to run ordinary errands like grocery shopping (which by the way, I never thought I'd actually miss pushing a creaky buggy down a brightly lit aisle squinting at my list of produce), or to even feel well enough to cook, clean, read a book, or watch TV. After 4 rounds of A.C., it was on to 12 rounds of Taxol, and thankfully, Taxol was much easier to tolerate. During chemo, the fatigue was the type that rivaled that of new motherhood.

Except now, I was the one who needed taking care of.

Chemo fatigue held me close to its bosom like a nursing infant, and I could do nothing to get free of it but sleep. I slept often because it was the only way I could escape the all-consuming nausea, and I just didn't have the energy to do anything else. There were days that I could barely make it to my bed before my body just shut down, and I'd be asleep for hours. Sleeping UnBeauty instead of Chemorella. Day 3 after my infusion, when the premedications began to wear off, was always the worst day for me. Although I did not throw up until closer to the end of my A.C. treatment, it was hard to find comfort in food because everything tasted horrible or "off", too bitter or too sweet, and my digestive system seemed to have come to a halt. Even water tasted bad. I would only drink out of glass cups because anything aluminum or plastic had a weird metallic aftertaste. My skin even smelled different to me. The subtle but medicinal smell of the chemo seemed to cling to me, seeping from my pores. I could no longer wear perfume or use scented lotion or soaps because the smell would add to my nausea. My skin and mouth were perpetually dry, and I began to have extreme night sweats. If my white blood cell count came back too low, I would have to receive a shot every single day for five days straight to help increase the numbers before I could have my next chemo. The shots would make my bones and joints ache like I'd run a marathon without stretching or without the physical fitness to actually participate in such a task. Again; so rude!

I remember there were a few times that I'd wake from a nausea-laced sleep to find my husband, Mike, standing at our bedroom doorway, his dark eyes full of concern, and then I'd drift back off, unable to stay awake or get up. Occasionally, my hand would rest over the edge of the mattress, and I'd feel Bear, my German Shepherd's cold, wet nose press against my open palm as if to say, "Come on, wake up! Why are you sleeping so much? Let's play!"

There were times that I sat slumped over on the living room couch, staring blindly off into the distance, praying for the nausea to subside. I felt like a zombie. So much of those weeks would go by in a blur. Did my family eat dinner those nights? Did my teenage son bathe regularly? Who knew! All I know is that I was a shadow of myself and it was one of the loneliest and darkest times of my life. Although my practical side knew that all of this was only temporary, at the time it did not feel like it. So engrossed in my nausea and inability to do more than slump around the house or sleep, I couldn't help but wonder if this was my new normal. I was under the impression that all 16 rounds of chemotherapy would feel like the equivalent of being hit head-on by a Mack truck whose driver was blind and in the throes of inexplicable road rage.

To add insult to injury was the helpless feeling that I was alone in this experience even though I knew that wasn't truly the case. I didn't know anyone else my age at that time who was battling breast cancer, and I felt that none of my friends could relate or empathize with what I was going through. If I heard one more person tell me that it was "just hair" and that it "would grow back," I thought that I would scream. Although ultimately, this was true, and it was meant to be reassuring and encouraging, I felt that I had lost a big piece of my identity, and besides, I didn't have the cheekbones for a pixie cut! Who am I? Natalie Portman? Not to mention the amount of time it would take to grow back.

I'd search videos on YouTube to try to help me understand if what I was going through was "normal." I consoled myself with the thought that if the chemo was making me feel this bad, then it meant that it was working and that even if it was killing all of the good cells (and maybe a little bit of my spirit in the process), then it was killing the cancer too. I would stare longingly at my husband, but not for lascivious reasons...I was jealous of his good cells. I'd watch him walk around all healthy and unbothered, thinking to myself, "Look at him, enjoying his youth and cancer-free cells." The audacity! My eyes narrowed and my mouth set to a grim line as the small violin played on in the background of my new existence and the nausea settled over every fiber of my body like a heavy cloak. This was reminiscent of the days when our children were babies, and I'd be awake rocking and nursing them at all hours of the night as he slumbered on in blissful oblivion. I'd sit across the dark room, staring daggers at him, thinking, "You did this to me!"

I was also very jealous of women with long, thick hair because I missed my own. I'd watch unabashedly while the subject of my envy would toss her hair over her shoulder or walk past with a bouncy ponytail trailing after her. I'd stare to the point that I probably creeped a few of them out. Here I was feeling like Golem from The Lord of the Rings, staring at women with their full heads of hair as I sat practically rubbing my hands together, muttering, "My precious..." in their direction.

But it wasn't all pain and suffering. During the recovery weeks (you get one week for your body to recover before the next A.C. infusion), I was reborn. I'd get my chemo on a Tuesday, and then by around Saturday, I'd wake feeling more like myself and less sick. I'd step outside and suddenly I'd be struck by the brilliance of the sun and how fresh the air was. I'd inhale deeply and blink rapidly like a baby fawn coming outside for the first time after a harsh winter. I was always so grateful for those recovery weeks, although they became shorter and shorter as each round stayed in my system a little longer. Another perk (but wait, there's more!) was that I also got a lot of unsolicited free meals because my friends, not knowing how to console me and wanting to express their support and love, would often buy me lunch or dinner. To this, I didn't complain and was also very grateful! Sometimes you have to let others help you heal.

As someone who has always been a caretaker to everyone else, it was very difficult for me to let others take care of me for a change. During this time, it brought me so much closer to my children, their dad, and my true friends. Nothing solidifies a bond like real vulnerability, empathy, compassion, and a deeper connection forged by something as delicate, complex, and unpredictable as a serious health concern. When you are in a more vulnerable position than you have ever been before, it is in these moments of weakness that help us create stronger relationships with God and with the people who matter most to us. This, in turn, actually becomes a strength. My good friend, Tammy Lynn, who is also a breast cancer survivor, once said to me, "You know how they say that it takes a village to raise a child? Well, cancer is the same way; it takes a village to beat cancer!" Cancer and chemo taught me not only to really appreciate my body and my health but to value the time I spent with the people around me—my village.

CHAPTER 8

While there's no way to know for certain which side effects one will or won't have during chemo; each battle is unique to the individual, there are a few tips and reminders I want to share that might help any aspiring Chemorellas.

When you have the energy, walk, do yoga, or find something low-impact that will keep your blood flowing and your muscles active. Check with your doctor if you're not sure what is safe. Not only does moving our bodies release good endorphins, but it helped me feel more in control of my health. In my opinion, the better shape you can be in, the easier it seems to recover.

Eat! Pretend that you have a persistent Filipino mother standing over your shoulder with a wooden spoon, urging you to eat even though later she will ruthlessly point out that you've gained weight. Eat meals like you usually would, but in smaller portions, even if you don't have much of an appetite. One of my nurses told me that eating regularly helps metabolize chemo, and this did seem to help me keep up more of my strength. Our bodies need good nutrients to heal, especially during chemo.

Take your medications on schedule. I resisted taking my anti-nausea medicine because I didn't want to take medicine, but once the nausea was at its peak, the medication didn't seem to be able to put a dent in how ill I felt, so it would have been better for me to stay on top of it and take it before the nausea was at its worst. It also helps to take your anti-diarrhea or constipation medication regularly (I had the joy of dealing with the latter of these two side effects).

Find a support group. Being able to talk to someone or to others who understand what you are going through will help you feel less alone and frightened. I have to be honest, I was afraid to join a breast cancer support group because I worried that seeing other women suffer, or worse, lose their battle, would only depress me further, but the friendships that I've made as a result of the breast cancer support groups that I've been a part of have helped me significantly. Surrounding myself with a sisterhood of strong, courageous, and loving women has made me love life even more and has given me more hope and confidence.

Let people help you. One thing I learned when I was in the fog of A.C. was that the world won't end without me. My kids learned to be more independent and empathetic while I was out of commission. And it brought me closer to my true friends who showed up for me and offered to bring meals, attend appointments, or anything else I might need help with. Asking for help is extremely hard for me, and I was lucky that my husband and kids were there to help out. I can only speak from the perspective of someone whose children were old enough to care for themselves, and my heart goes out to all the mommas with infants or young children to care for, some as single parents while they are going through chemo. Most hospitals have navigators who can help connect you to resources and local organizations. This is another reason a support group is helpful; because you may learn about so many useful things you may never have even heard of through the women who can speak from experience and who know others who can help. And again, who cares if there are some dishes in the sink or some laundry that hasn't been folded yet? It's not a big deal, and your family will learn to step up more and become caregivers themselves.

Speaking of friends, focus on the ones who are there, not the ones who stopped calling or texting during chemo. Sometimes it's not even about us, and that person may be going through their own personal fire at the same time as ours and just cannot be available emotionally. And while it'd be nice for them to communicate this, if they don't, don't waste the energy you so desperately need to help heal yourself in the absence of someone who has made themselves scarce during this time in your life. A friend of mine revealed later that she never asked me about my cancer treatment because she was afraid that it would only upset me or make me sad. I had interpreted this as her indifference, and while I didn't want a pity party, it had caused me to disengage in our friendship until I later understood her reasoning a little better. It was hard for me to go from being the one who always checked on everyone else to the one who was deeply struggling and who did not know how to fully open up. Finding the right support systems, being honest and communicative, and spending time with my friends and family throughout my treatment when I was able to made a big difference in my healing process.

Find a good alcohol-free mouthwash. I used mouthwash nightly and I think this might have helped prevent mouth sores. Sucking on mints might also help with the dry mouth. Ask your doctor when in doubt.

Keep a diary of your symptoms day to day. This will help you see any patterns with your health, and it will help you keep track of side effects or issues that you may need to discuss with your doctor. It's essential that you advocate for yourself as much as possible and be very upfront with what you may be experiencing mentally and emotionally as well as physically. Keeping a journal also helped me process some of my emotions and allowed me to look back at everything I experienced and learned.

Keep going and be patient with yourself. Never lose hope, and do not feel guilty for prioritizing yourself.

You are beautiful. Post-chemo Golem look alike or not.

CHAPTER 9

Life after 6 long, grueling months of chemo was a strange dichotomy of emotions. On the one hand, I was happy to be done with the infusions! I was so eager for my hair to grow back. My precious... and to my surprise, it began growing back slowly during the last rounds of Taxol, most of it coming in white and gray and a bit wavy, but it was back. With it came a glimmer of the old Emily that I so desperately wanted to see and know again.

I can forgive my body for not having the melanin to produce black, shiny hair instead of the crinkly gray stuff that was sprouting across my scalp since my body was also working so hard to restore me to default settings. I remember being so excited about the new peach fuzz, even though, to my disdain, it was only growing on the sides of my head and not on the top, so I spent the first few months looking like Mr. Burns from The Simpsons. Watch out, world! Momma has a new look!

On one occasion, my dear mother, the strongest woman I know, who is also a breast cancer survivor (so you'd think she'd have been a little more sympathetic to my plight), came to visit me. She came bearing food, so of course, I ushered her in. I wore a knitted cap around the house to keep my head warm, and I excitedly pulled the cap off to show her my new hair—male pattern baldness and all—to which she gasped at the sight of my new do and loudly exclaimed, "Is it going to stay like that?!" I chuckle thinking of how quickly I jammed my cap back on under her harsh but comical scrutiny. Ah, mothers, the source of all our insecurities! How is it that moms can be so critical and innocuous all at the same time? I owe so much to my mother, Evelyn. She never really talked much about her own breast cancer diagnosis until much later, and as with so many things, I see now how much she faced and endured with an impressive amount of grace and dignity.

After chemo was complete, I was also, of course, thrilled to be done poisoning my body and ruining the "good cells" that I so coveted. Praise God, the chemo did its job! The results of my scan had shown no evidence of cancer, and the tumor in my breast shrunk to the point that it was undetectable!

Aside from that, I'd also be able to taste my food again and not feel so worn out and tired. I could picture myself taking my dog on long jogs again and losing some of the chemo weight I put on due to the steroids. I was so ready to get back to being me.

But on the other hand, one question seemed to plague me: What did that version of me even look and behave like now?

I was not the same woman I was 6 months prior, and not just physically. Although I didn't like going to chemotherapy, I made good friendships with the nurses on the oncology floor, and there was some comfort and safety in having a set routine. With my chemotherapy complete, I'd be moving full speed ahead to the next scary phases: surgery and then radiation. During the treatment part of my diagnosis, everything was planned out by my team of doctors. All I had to do was show up. But now, I'd have to navigate fully recovering from all of the chemo without the nurses who I considered my support squad being around me each week to guide me. It was bittersweet—a milestone that was also a goodbye.

I returned to work during Taxol, and while it was a struggle, I was glad to have some form of normalcy, but this version of myself who returned to work was different from the version of myself who used to be an overachiever. That old version showed up for everyone else; that one had the stamina and confidence to push herself to achieve her goals...this new Emily...she was a little bit of a stranger and she felt tired and weak. She still felt alone. I had yet to join a support group or find other women my age recovering from cancer, so I was uncertain of what was or wasn't "normal" to feel.

I was still wearing wigs occasionally, and sometimes I felt as though I was just impersonating myself. Honestly, I was afraid that I wouldn't be as good as I was before I got cancer. When everyone hears that you're done with treatment, they are quick to think, "Okay, great! Back to the regularly scheduled program now that you're all healed!" But they didn't understand that while I did not want pity, nor did I want cancer to define me, I was still grappling with how to reclaim all that was taken from me. My identity, for one. The scariest of all questions was how do I overcome the fear of recurrence? How do I continue to move up in my demanding job as I had planned when all I wanted to do was lay on the couch and sleep? Am I still good enough to take on all of these responsibilities and projects that came along with a fairly new role? Would I have the energy and the self-confidence to be a leader or to attend all these meetings and not cry unexpectedly when something reminded me of how different I felt? Am I going to have the mental and emotional bandwidth to be the best mother, partner, friend, daughter, sister, or employee that I was before? All of the unanswerable questions felt daunting and if I could give my fresh-from-chemo self some advice, I'd tell myself to stop worrying so much and to just be. It's okay not to have it all figured out, and it's okay not to feel like your old self. Don't be afraid of letting others down or not being strong enough or good enough because at the end of the day, the fact that you are still here and still making the most out of life says a lot. Just put one foot in front of the other and give yourself the time, patience, and grace to just be in the here and now. There is no finish line to being "normal" again after chemo. Sometimes we feel more emotional months or even years after our treatment, and that's okay too. What's important is how we take care of ourselves and how we protect our mental, physical, and emotional well-being throughout the process. There is no linear way to heal from any kind of trauma, big or small, especially when cancer is involved.

Getting through lingering side effects is another hurdle that takes patience. Chemo fog is a real thing. Much like "mommy brain," I felt like my focus and memory weren't quite the same as before. I often struggled to find the words to the most common of things, like "cabinet." I became frustrated and exasperated when my husband didn't understand exactly what I meant when I made requests like, "Grab me a can of vegetables out of the 'thingy.' You know! The thing! The one place with the stuff inside!"

I was worried that in addition to chemo fog, after being under anesthesia six times (one surgery to insert my medi-port for chemo and then five major surgeries, a complete hysterectomy due to BRCA2 being one of them) all in a little over a year, I wasn't as 'sharp' as I was prior to my treatments. I didn't want my coworkers to feel as though I couldn't handle the pressure or workload of my position and that I needed special treatment or accommodations, even though there's nothing to be ashamed of when it comes to needing help or reasonable accommodations at work. I was very blessed to have a great team and manager who offered so much support and encouragement.

Another thing that I was still struggling with was my body and self-image. Whenever I saw myself undressed, this scarred, misshapen chested woman looked back at me. I felt amputated and like my youth and fertility were stripped from me. I never completed my breast reconstruction as planned. I opted to get chest expanders, which are like temporary breast implants that help stretch the skin in the chest area enough to where breast implants could then eventually be placed. The skin on my left breast began to "die" and the skin in that area grew so thin that the expander began to come through it. This all began to happen seemingly out of nowhere and with no real explanation that the doctors could offer. Thankfully, even though the expander could literally be seen protruding from my chest, the skin surrounding it didn't hurt because I didn't appear to have enough nerve endings in that area so recently after my bilateral mastectomy, but it had to be removed and debrided. Unfortunately, it happened a second time on the same side two weeks later and when it did, I advised my plastic surgeon to remove the expander altogether and let me heal for several months with the intention to revisit reconstruction at a later date. It was all incredibly overwhelming and the surgeries were painful, leaving me sore, tender, and unable to sleep on my side for many weeks.

I reminded myself that while having breasts is a big part of being feminine, it's not what makes me a woman. I was blessed and grateful to be alive, and as a result, I threw myself into opening a boutique for breast cancer patients called The Boobie Boutique. I wanted to help other women who have gone through many of the same struggles that I experienced during my fight with cancer. My wish was to take all of the sadness, fear, and suffering and turn it into something beautiful. A safe haven and a place to help rebuild one's self-esteem and confidence after chemotherapy and surgery. Starting The Boobie Boutique was one of the hardest but one of the best experiences of my life, and I can safely say that if it weren't for my cancer journey and all of the ups and downs of chemotherapy, I may never have realized my passion and true calling to become a mastectomy bra and wig fitter.

Like many people, before I was diagnosed with cancer, I was under the impression that by removing my breasts and the source of the cancer, I could go about the rest of my life not having to worry about it ever again. I didn't realize that's not exactly how it works, and that after any cancer diagnosis, you are now living with a possible recurrence looming over you. With each scan, the fear and anxiety of bad results will bloom in the dark corners of your mind and settle in your heart like a ticking bomb. Each little cough or ache will send alarm bells going off. Is it cancer? Has it returned? And if it has returned, is it back with a vengeance? The anxiety and internal battle are potent, and it's torturous waiting the week or however long it takes to get the results. After my most recent CT scan, I burst into tears after reading the results online. So huge was my relief that the cancer had not returned in my brain, lungs, liver, or anywhere else. There is no easy way to manage these fears that I have discovered, but I will say that I continue to trust in God and do the work to redirect my thoughts as much as possible and find good distractions and activities that I enjoy to help ease the "scanxiety," as they call it. I make the choice every day not to worry over the things that I have no control over, and just like the first time, I know He is there and will always be, along with my family and friends, if cancer were to return. Living in fear only diminishes your ability to truly and fully enjoy the time that you have right now.

As morbid as it sounds, I did ask myself what I would do if the cancer came back for me in 5 years. What would I want to do with my life and who would I want to become if there was a good possibility that I would not live long enough to grow old? The answer to those questions was that I didn't just want to exist. I wanted to live as boldly and fearlessly as possible and that meant doing everything that scared me, including starting a business and leaping headfirst into the unknown. I left my cushy corporate job and decided that after everything that I went through and was still going through, I owed it to myself to find my true passion and to build something that was truly fulfilling, and that is another reason that The Boobie Boutique was born.

I'd like to think that when something really hard happens to us in life and a piece of us dies in the process, this is the time when God brings the best parts of Him out in us. We don't always have a choice but to be strong and to be brave, but we do have a choice to re-emerge brand new, even stronger, wiser, and more grateful and joyful than before. Every deep struggle, every setback, and every loss has a lesson and a new beginning with the potential for a powerful outcome.

I've had the massive pleasure and extreme honor of meeting many other breast cancer survivors who have faced so much, cancer sometimes only being the tip of the iceberg, and yet they haven't shrunk away from life. They haven't allowed cancer to destroy their effervescent spirits or minimize them as people. Cancer robbed them, hurt them, and even broke them at times, but they rose like a phoenix, and not only did they rise, they held out their hands to the sister battling next to them and helped lift her up too.

In many ways, I feel as though my life truly began after I was diagnosed with ER & PR+ stage II invasive ductal carcinoma in October of 2021. I'm proud of the woman I have become and am still evolving into. I have gained more wisdom and have truly begun learning to love myself more, as well as cherishing self-care. It is with awe and gratitude that I can say that since I completed chemo in April of 2022, I haven't had a cold or been ill since. I can run 3 miles without exhausting myself. I dance like no one is watching when the songs of my youth come on the radio (give me the 90s and early 2000s hits any day). I take so much pleasure in the little things in life. Feeling the wind blowing in my hair with the windows rolled down as I'm driving down the highway, listening to music makes me breathe in deeply and with a resounding sense of gratitude. Here I am. I live not only for myself and for my family but for my sisters who fought so hard but couldn't be here today. I look for opportunities to do the things that scare me but that I know will develop my character or teach me something new, because let's face it, I already went through one of the scariest things that I could imagine. Nothing, not even public speaking, failure, or possibly making a fool of myself in front of others, is that scary anymore. There is something liberating about knowing that you are truly brave even if you had no choice but to be.

Life after chemo is a rebirth. It's a testimony of God's strength and love. It's a reflection of the resilience of the human spirit and of His glory. Rebuilding your life after chemo and cancer is a love story to yourself, a translation of fear and pain turned into hope and strength. It's a love story because cancer changes the way that you perceive time and life; it makes many of us really want to take better care of ourselves and prioritize the things that make us happy. Loss is cancer's muse, and while it may be true what they say about not knowing what you have until it's gone, you also don't know what's possible within yourself until you have learned to let go.

I've lost a few friends over the past couple of years, and this is never easy. You see yourself in these women. You know how much they loved their families and how much they had to give to the world. They were filled with unique experiences and dreams. They loved to live, laugh, and love, as the popular home décor signs would say. You know that they smiled even when they were afraid or in pain. That they probably cried in the shower or into their pillows while everyone else was asleep because they didn't want to upset their families or wanted others to see how frightened or sad they were. You know because you have done it too. You are her and she is you. The injustice of it all, of the world losing a mother, a sister, an aunt, a daughter, a wife, a friend, and a warrior is heartbreaking and infuriating. You know that it could just as easily be you. This is why I feel it's so important to be present in life as much as possible. We honor them by living with more—living with more love, more compassion, more hope, more excitement, more trust, more Jesus, more everything.

—Emily Hardin

TINA'S STORY

CHAPTER 10

My breast cancer story begins in September of 2008. My husband and I had been married for 20 years, and we had never really had any vacations that didn't involve going to see family. In 2006, my husband lost his mind and opened a pizzeria. We'd been working six days a week since April 15, 2006, and I was exhausted! I needed a break.

I was able to plan a quick getaway from California to Niagara Falls for our 20th wedding anniversary over Labor Day weekend in 2008. It was there that our lives would be forever changed.

We arrived on Friday of Labor Day weekend. That night was gorgeous with the Northern Lights—breathtaking! On Saturday, as I was getting out of the shower, I bent over to dry off and noticed that my left breast's nipple was slightly inverted. When I stood back up, it went back to normal. I bent back over, and it inverted again.

My gut told me that I had breast cancer. I was devastated, and at that moment, I got back in the shower and cried. When I got back out and was drying off again, it happened again. It wasn't my imagination. How I wished it was! I was numb, yet at the same time, I was overcome with emotion. I didn't want to ruin my trip for myself or my husband in this beautiful location, especially with our hotel room overlooking Niagara Falls. The lights on Niagara Falls and the Northern Lights the night before were breathtaking.

I kept those things in my mind and continued on my day, sightseeing and enjoying life with my husband, knowing that when I got home, I would have some testing and some hard decisions to make. But at that moment, I was determined to enjoy life. I made a conscious decision not to tell my husband anything at that time, as I wanted him to enjoy our much-needed and long-awaited vacation/honeymoon together. We didn't get one 20 years ago.

There were times throughout that Saturday and into that evening that I wanted to go back home, but then I remembered that it was a holiday, so even if I cut our trip short and went home, I couldn't get a doctor's appointment on Monday, as everything would be closed. So I put on my happy, brave face and continued on; it's what I had done so many times throughout my life.

Once home, a little bit of denial set in, as I didn't make my appointment as soon as I returned home. I had fires to put out at work, and things happened while we were gone that we had to deal with. It was a great distraction, actually! I just put the possibility of breast cancer in the back of my mind. I was 41 years old. I had a mammogram in April, and breast cancer didn't run in my family. I didn't realize I had any risk factors. I have since found out that I did but wasn't aware at the time.

I waited two weeks to call my doctor. I went to see my PCP, who did a breast exam and made an urgent referral to my OB-GYN so that I could have another breast exam, and my OB-GYN could then order a mammogram. I didn't ask why he couldn't order it; I just went with what he said at the time. I got an appointment for the last week of September 2006 with a brand new OB-GYN who had never seen me before. The doctor walked in with a student physician doing clinicals. She asked me if I minded if the student did my exam.

With my sense of humor, I said, "Yes, that's fine, but you're going to do it first or second—I don't care which way you do it, but you're also going to do it." She was kind of confused as to why I wanted a double exam. They had scheduled me for a physical. Once I explained to her that I had nipple inversion, she completely understood my concerns and I requested that she also do the exam alongside the student.

The student felt around and didn't feel anything. The doctor felt around and discovered something. The doctor had the student feel again, but the student still couldn't feel anything. So the doctor put her hand over the student's hand and guided it to the exact placement of what my doctor was feeling. The student said, "Oh, OK—now I feel that." A mammogram was ordered stat and was actually done two hours later. I was then scheduled for a left and a right ultrasound-assisted breast biopsy.

To my dismay, they refused to do both biopsies on the same day, giving me some excuse that it was uncomfortable for the patient and that they just don't do that. So, in the very first week of October, I had the left biopsy done. I was fine. I could have had the other side done, but nope. The second week, I had the right biopsy done. Back then, there was no electronic access to my chart, so I waited. While I waited, I made an appointment with the surgeon. I talked to his nurse—not the front desk person. I explained what was going on and she gave me two appointments: one was the initial consultation, but she also put me on her surgery schedule for a lumpectomy for October 31, 2006.

I had an appointment with my new OB-GYN to get my results. She walked in with a very gloomy look on her face. She told me, "I'm so sorry to tell you, but you have breast cancer." I replied, "I know; I already have made an appointment with my surgeon." She then looked confused and moved closer to me. She took both hands, put them gently on my cheeks, and said, "I don't think you understand what I said. I just told you, you have breast cancer." She was slightly emotional as she told me.

I then responded, "I understand what you said, but you didn't tell me I have leukemia, which both my parents passed away from. I have breast cancer, so let's take them off, put them back on, and I'm good." She kind of giggled at that and then asked me why I brought up leukemia.

I said, "Oh, you didn't read my family history; both of my parents passed away eight months apart from AML leukemia. In my experience, leukemia has a 0% survival rate, and breast cancer, I feel like I have a 50-50 shot. So although I'm not happy with breast cancer, given my parents' history, I feel it's the lesser of two evils. I know I have no choice in what I've got."

After that appointment, I had to go home and have what I thought at the time was going to be one of the hardest conversations I've had to have with my husband and my three kids. I hadn't said much about it throughout the testing and all. My husband, when told, went into a very deep depression. It was extremely hard to watch. He heard the words "breast cancer," and even though I told him I was going to be fine, his world fell apart, and he acted as if I was dying.

CHAPTER 11

Our youngest daughter was the only one still home at the time; she had just turned 15. Telling her was harder than telling my husband. As her mom, I wanted to protect her and make her world "OK," and I couldn't. Instead, I was the one hurting her, and knowing this was so hard on me was, in some ways, harder than the cancer diagnosis. My mom passed away in December of 2000; she was only 54, and although my daughter was only in first or second grade when that happened, Grandma was her best friend; my mom was my little girl's world. Now I was telling my daughter that her mom had cancer. Everybody she's ever known at that point that had cancer had passed away. Instead of drawing closer to me, she pushed away and got further away. That was so hard. I felt helpless and had nowhere to turn for guidance on how to help her or reach her.

I then had to call our oldest two daughters—one was in the Army and one was in the Navy. I had to tell my other two daughters that I had breast cancer over the phone instead of in person, which was not the way I wanted to do it, but with them being in the military, I didn't really have a choice. Zoom wasn't "a thing" in 2008, and neither was FaceTime.

We owned a pizzeria, and we were in the process of moving to a larger location where we were buying the building. I wanted to stop that process, and another part of me wanted to carry on, as stopping the process felt like giving in to my cancer, and I felt like, at that time, the cancer would have won. It was already taking my breasts; I didn't want it to take anything else. Boy, was I naïve to all that was about to come.

I met with my surgeon four days before I was scheduled for surgery. He walked in to do the consultation and was pretty confused by what had happened. I wasn't sure what to say, and honestly, I don't remember what I said, but I believe I blamed it on my primary care physician having something to do with the scheduling. I know I didn't want to get his nurse in trouble for scheduling me that way.

During my consultation, it was confirmed that I had invasive ductal carcinoma in my left breast and lobular carcinoma in my right breast. I had wanted a mastectomy; however, I couldn't get my plastic surgeon and my surgeon together on the same day to do it at the same time. I agreed to just do a lumpectomy. I just wanted the cancer out of me RIGHT NOW!! However, I wasn't happy about a lumpectomy, and I had a long talk with God. I asked God that if I was making the wrong decision by having a lumpectomy versus a mastectomy, let them not get clear margins or something happen that makes it crystal clear to all involved that I need a mastectomy, not another lumpectomy. I can say without a doubt: be careful what you ask for...

On the day of surgery, I had to be at the hospital at 5:30 AM for a 7:00 AM surgery. My husband and I arrived and in the waiting room sat a customer from our pizzeria on her laptop. She looked up as I walked in the door and said, "Piser, you're late." I replied, "I'm not late! I'm right on time. That means you're late; you should have been here 15 minutes ago." Although I didn't know her except from the pizzeria, I felt so much support, relief that she was there, and love from her that day, which continues on to this day. At that moment, Robin was the friend I didn't know I had.

I was taken back for surgery prep, and after that, I remember nothing until around 4:00 or 5:00 the next morning. I woke up in a hospital room trying to figure out what time of day it was. I could see a clock on the wall, but I couldn't find my glasses to see the time. My room was dark and the door was closed. I had a blood pressure cuff on my right arm and something squeezing my legs, and that was what woke me up. There was nobody in my room. I had to turn the TV on to see what was on to try and determine whether it was 4:00 PM or 4:00 AM the next day. Sure enough, it was 4:00 AM, November 1st, and at that point, I was very confused because my lumpectomy was supposed to be a very easy, simple surgery. I was supposed to go home the same day.

I buzzed for the nurse, and she came in and said something like, "Oh, sleeping beauty is finally awake." Haha. She brought me some apple juice and crackers and didn't tell me much, just that the doctor would be in to see me as he made rounds. A few hours went by that seemed like forever, and then my surgeon came in and explained what happened. I had a violent reaction to coming out of the anesthesia. I was very sick; I was throwing up, my blood pressure was fluctuating, and they gave me fluids, but I wouldn't wake up properly, so he had to put me upstairs instead of allowing me to go home.

Next, he went on to tell me that my right side, with the lobular cancer, was lobular in situ stage 0 but also had in situ ductal carcinoma. The left side was invasive ductal carcinoma stage 2. The right sentinel node was clear, but the left sentinel node was cancerous. They took out a cluster of 18, and eleven of them contained cancer. Then, he informed me that on the left side, they did not get clear margins, and due to a complication, I would need to make the choice of a single or a double mastectomy, as going back in to do a lumpectomy was no longer an option.

He explained to me that when he went to excise the tumor on the left side, the whole breast fell apart, and he had to put it back together and sew me up. I guess my facial expression said it all with this information, as he then told me that once the bandages came off, it would look like a normal breast, but it would not feel like it when I touched it. There were no margins to go back in and re-excise.

Along with my breasts falling apart, my left arm was above my head for approximately a six-and-a-half-hour surgery. Due to the complication, I ended up with a frozen shoulder. Physical therapy was started and then stopped while I was scheduled for a mastectomy, then restarted. It took a total of 4 to 5 months to regain 50% range of motion. The rest was up to me. It took over a year, but I regained it.

Remember I said to be careful what you ask of God? He definitely answered me! Who's breast falls apart on the table having a mastectomy? Mine! Lol. I also try telling doctors that I am "special" or "complicated" when it comes to medical things, as I tend to have the "rare" side effects or complications, but until they experience it firsthand, they don't believe me.

I told my surgeon that I wanted to do a double mastectomy and asked him when we could do it? I knew I had to heal from one surgery before another. He knew who my plastic surgeon was and that I wanted him, and they had already consulted after my surgery. They came up with a date of December 10, 2008—perfect timing! My mom was diagnosed with AML on December 10, 1999.

The mastectomy surgery was uneventful. When the anesthesiologist came in to talk to me about the surgery, I explained to him what happened last time and asked him to pull my chart so that he could see what they gave me last time, in hopes that we could adjust the doses or something so that it wouldn't happen again.

He left, came back, and we talked about what I was given. He decided to use something completely different and a lower dose. I came out of my double mastectomy surgery just fine. I think I was in recovery for 3 to 4 hours, went upstairs to my room for the night, and was then discharged to go home after the surgeon came in to talk with me about the pathology.

Pathology on my mastectomy revealed another small invasive ductal carcinoma tumor on the left side that had not been detected in the mammogram or ultrasound. Needless to say, I was very happy with the decision to have a double mastectomy upon receiving that news! When would it have been found had the lumpectomy given clean margins? God was definitely in control!

My reconstruction surgery was started during the time I had my mastectomy with expanders. To be completely transparent and honest, had I known the pain I would be in and the discomfort of having the expanders in, I probably would not have agreed to do it. After the fact, I'm very happy that I did it, and I have no regrets!

Had someone told me that stretching the skin to expand it felt like bricks in my chest—where I felt like I could knock someone out if I moved just right and hit them in the head—I would have declined the procedure and opted to remain flat. I'm glad I was naïve at the time, thinking it wouldn't be much different from a boob job. Boy, was I WRONG! However, the exchange surgery was great!

My plastic surgeon expanded me on the day of surgery. The pain was excruciating, and I'm allergic to most pain medications. I had him remove some of the saline to give me time to heal from the surgery. He wasn't happy, as he wasn't understanding what was causing me so much pain in one spot—and on the right side only. It turned out to be the end of an internal stitch poking my skin. Once it dissolved, the pain vanished.

I never realized just how much I used my chest muscles until the expanders were under them. Lifting a glass was painful. I couldn't unscrew a 7-Up or water bottle for a few weeks. When my doctor said no lifting over five pounds, at first I thought, "Hmm, really? That little?" As I moved my arm, I understood why—and I couldn't have lifted 10 pounds if I tried.

CHAPTER 11

Every day, prior to leaving in the morning, my husband poured red solo cups of juice and water and put them on a shelf in the fridge that I could reach. He lowered everything I might want to eat, as I wasn't allowed to raise my arms past straight out in front of me. I used paper plates and plastic cutlery—not only for weight restrictions but also for clean-up.

This was all such an emotional time. My best friend of 10 to 11 years deserted me during this period. She hardly ever texted or called. I was devastated but didn't have the emotional bandwidth to deal with it. My friend Robin, who showed up at the hospital during my first surgery, texted me or stopped by the pizzeria at least once a week to check on how I was doing. My youngest daughter was rarely there. That hurt the most, but she was going through a lot too. I didn't know how to help her.

I declined chemotherapy. In doing so, my oncologist dismissed me as his patient for "non-compliance." My reason was simple: they only offered me chemotherapy that had a chance of causing AML later in life.

He dismissed my concerns about my family history with AML. I had a double mastectomy, and they stated no radiation was needed. I felt like I could return to my prior life before cancer. Again, how naïve. We are forever changed. I needed to mourn my previous life, but it was years before I realized that.

I had less patience for drama and nonsense. My husband disliked the rain. One day after my surgery, he came home mad—over rain?? Seriously?? Get out of here with that nonsense! I'm here recovering from having my breasts cut off, and you're pissed off it's raining outside? He realized how insignificant that was compared to what I was dealing with, and we both laughed.

I was missing work daily since October 31; I think I returned full-time in March 2009. Missing work was more than just work; it was also missing seeing and spending time with our youngest as she was there six days a week after school until close.

After I healed from my mastectomy and as I was going through the reconstruction process, I never looked at myself in the mirror. It took me almost four years to stand in front of a mirror and look at myself naked. I had seen pictures from others who had mastectomies, and I was terrified to look at myself. How did I manage that, you might ask? When I was in the shower, I dried off in the shower, wrapped the towel around me, went into my bedroom, and into my walk-in closet where there were no mirrors, and got dressed.

When I finally had the courage to look at myself, I was pleasantly surprised at my scar line. I had used emu oil on my scar while I was healing for about 8 weeks. I'm not sure if that had anything to do with it or not, but my scar line is very faint and looks almost like stretch marks.

Fast forward to Mother's Day 2010. I found a lump in my mastectomy scar line on the left side—all the way at the very end of the scar line towards my side. Throughout those past 18 months, as the weather would change, my new breasts became my weather vanes. If it was going to rain, they'd itch more than usual about 4 to 5 days before it rained. If it was warm and we were going to get a cold front moving in, they'd itch 4 to 5 days in advance. I was very familiar with how they felt. When I felt a lump, my "gut feeling" was the same as back 18 months prior: cancer again! It felt very tiny, oblong, hard, and felt like a grain of rice under my skin.

I went to my PCP because I could get in fastest with him. He felt it and said it was probably scar tissue. Not satisfied! I went to my oncologist, and he also said it was probably scar tissue. The hair on the back of my neck was standing up; my intuition was screaming at me, but I wasn't being taken seriously! I was mad but determined to be heard and taken seriously. I called my plastic surgeon and asked to be seen. He felt it, and although he said, "Probably scar tissue," he added, "But if I'm your third doctor you're seeing, let's take it out and get it biopsied." FINALLY, I was being heard!

A few days later, he removed the lump in the office. He showed it to me; it looked like normal scar tissue but was sent off to pathology. Two days later, I got a call—the doctor wanted me to come in for my results. Could I come now? Yes! I was at work and told my husband I was going to the doctor for the results.

Our daughter overheard that, took my keys, and said, "I'm driving!" Up until that point, she thought I was being dramatic and didn't believe it was back.

She's been around medicine her whole life, as Grandma was a nurse, and before the restaurant, I worked in a hospital lab. She knows that when results aren't given over the phone, it's usually not good news.

The doctor apologized as he felt he gave me false hope when he said it looked like "normal healthy scar tissue." He thought it was, but the cancer was embedded inside the scar tissue he removed. When pathology sliced it to make slides, it was seen—and it was invasive ductal carcinoma again! I wasn't expecting my reaction; when he said the words, I lost it. The entire way there, I was preparing myself and told myself to hold it together in front of my daughter—to be strong so she would worry less. That did NOT happen. What happened was I was a blubbering, crying mess, and my daughter ended up consoling me. It didn't last long, as I pulled it "back together." Boy, did I need my mom at this moment, yet I was glad she wasn't here. Watching her daughter go through cancer would have broken her heart just as it would mine if any of my three daughters received a cancer diagnosis.

A new oncologist was necessary because I didn't trust the other one. I did make an appointment with him before firing him to tell him off for dismissing my concerns and acting as if he had X-ray vision and could see inside me without a scan, ultrasound, or surgery consult! If I'd listened to him, would it have been found? Where would it have gone?

My new oncologist listened to my concerns about the risk of AML down the line from chemotherapy. We agreed on a type of chemo that doesn't carry that risk. I forget what we used, but I researched it and talked to my mom's oncologist about it over the phone, and he assured me it was okay. He was two hours away, or he would have been my doctor. I needed someone closer if possible. I had four infusions. I didn't do a port; I wish I had, as my veins in my hand are now damaged from the chemo.

I was so exhausted from chemotherapy. My brain didn't work right. I couldn't remember the simplest of things. I wasn't aware, but I was out of it the first 7 to 10 days. My youngest took me to each chemo appointment and sat with me while I was infused. I think she read, and I believe I slept. Honestly, I don't know. What I "thought I knew" about those four months isn't reality, as both my husband and daughter say I was a hot mess, and not good at all. They don't elaborate. It's okay, as it was traumatic for them, and I'm oblivious. Asking about it makes them relive it, so I don't.

We had a large German Shepherd; he weighed 120 pounds, all muscle and fur. I recall feeling good one afternoon, so I decided to take the dog for a walk. Huge mistake!! I walked across the street and down two to three houses (each 1 to 1.5 acres) and sat on the curb. I was winded and weak. I took my phone with me and had to call my husband to come get me. He was 15 minutes away at the pizzeria. I felt dumb and embarrassed to have to have him leave to come get me to take me basically across the street back home. He wasn't mad; he was scared and concerned.

A doctor appointment a few days later confirmed my counts were extremely low—not quite at needing a transfusion but very close. I was now "grounded." My daughter took my car and keys. It was summer, and I was freezing cold! I slept with a heated blanket on; I was so cold. Normally I'm hot when I sleep. I was on the couch once again for four months due to being freezing cold from low counts. The things they don't tell you!

Radiation was next. Oh boy! I remember all of that! I made a comment about how easy chemo was compared to radiation, and my daughter asked me what drugs I was on to think that and said I was very wrong.

I underwent 72 rounds of radiation, ended up with second-degree burns, and experienced worse fatigue than I recalled from chemotherapy. Chemo fatigue kept me tired all day and I felt the need to sleep all the time. Radiation fatigue would hit me out of nowhere. I could be going about my day at work, and it would feel like I hit a brick wall—I would need a nap right then and there! Two hours later, I was good to go again for the rest of the night.

When the machine broke down right after I'd had a week off to let my skin heal a little, I was given an extra week off; it was pure bliss for those two weeks! My last radiation day was Christmas Eve, 2010. It took me almost five months to regain my stamina and energy level after radiation.

CHAPTER 12

On Thanksgiving Day in November 2011, I woke up in a pool of blood. Off to the ER we went. I hadn't had a period since chemo in June 2010. I was 44 at this point. They did an emergency D&C to stop the bleeding, and the doctor told me I needed a hysterectomy; his office would be in contact with me. I had uterine pre-cancerous cells.

The hysterectomy was scheduled for December 6, 2011. Happy 45th to me!! As I was coming out of anesthesia, they administered additional pain meds through my IV—and I coded. If I am not allergic, I'm a toddler for doses! They don't "listen."

I just don't do things "normally"!

The biopsy revealed only pre-cancerous cells, so no further treatment was needed. Praise the Lord for that! They wanted me on Tamoxifen in 2008, but just the thought of it after I read the side effects, including "possible uterine cancer," made me refuse to take it. Every fiber of my being screamed no. I didn't take it, but had pre-cancerous cells. I dodged a bullet by listening to my body; otherwise, I might have had another cancer to deal with. Breast cancer twice, 18 months apart, was enough!

After having breast cancer twice so very close together, I started more research on it. I didn't "appear" to have risk factors, yet here I was. I was looking for answers to see if there possibly was one.

I found out that I had two second cousins (sisters) who, in 2011-2012, were in their early to mid-70s and had breast cancer back when they were 45 to 50 years of age. They were my grandfather's (on my mother's side) sister's daughters. My grandfather is 1 of 11 kids, and they are the only two out of all the siblings and their kids to have had it. As of 2024, both are still cancer-free and living their best lives in Havasu. Not a risk, as they are too far removed in the gene line.

After my diagnosis, my father's sister was diagnosed in 2011. That was not really a risk, as it was not on my mother's side, I was told.

What I did have was a history of birth control for 9 to 10 years, dense breast tissue, and fibrocystic breasts. Ding, ding, ding...risk factors. From the time I was 14 or 15 until I was 35 years old, I'd had 1 to 3 cysts drained via fine needle aspiration per year. Most of those cysts were in the left breast, which is the same breast where the invasive ductal carcinoma was found.

In 2016, we closed our business and sold the building to avoid bankruptcy. I wish I could blame it all on breast cancer, but I can't. It had a lot to do with it. We had also made mistakes, and those, along with being away from the business during my cancer and who we left in charge in our absence, caused too much damage to recover from.

It was a blessing in disguise, as we then moved out of California for financial reasons to Florida, where we could afford to live and rebuild our life in January 2017. For the first time in my 50 years of living, I was in a brand-new state.

Moving here was emotionally HARD, as I left my youngest daughter in California. Now an adult and on her own, she will always be my baby. We had been through a lot together, and it broke my heart to leave and be so far away, but financially we couldn't stay.

It ended up being best for my health, although I had no idea of that at the time.

Once in Florida, I returned to my previous profession as a medical lab assistant/phlebotomist. Honestly, after ten years in the restaurant industry, I was over dealing with rude customers who disrespected people in the service industry. Not all of them, of course. I'm not sure if it was where we were located or what, but there were enough rude customers. I kicked several out of the restaurant; no one disrespects my staff or myself.

They'd tell me, "I know the owner" when something wasn't right, or I said no to a request that I knew would back up my kitchen due to how we did things or, the worst was: "No ID, no beer." I'd just laugh and say, "Well, I guess you should step outside and call them then if you know them."

A lot of customers thought I was "just an employee," as I worked the front end just like everyone else and I looked "young," so I couldn't have been the owner. Lol.

In the medical profession, patients can be difficult, but that's okay! They're sick and feel terrible. They get a pass for a poor attitude, especially when I'm going to be sticking them with a needle to draw blood. I truly loved my patients and my job.

In 2017, I established a relationship with an oncologist here in Florida. In California, I'd been moved to yearly follow-up and a "call if you need us" type of thing. Here, he said, "No. Your cancer returned in a short time. You then had cervical pre-cancer. You will be seen every three months as a new patient. After two years, if all goes well, you'll be seen every six months." Sounds good to me!

CHAPTER 13

By late June 2020, I started experiencing a bronchial-sounding cough. I'm asthmatic, and it sounded and felt similar. COVID was happening, and I was in a mask for 7 to 8 hours a day, so asthma seemed a reasonable explanation. Breast cancer was not on my radar! I worked at COVID testing sites and vaccine sites, so I was tested often and was clear of COVID and the flu.

By late July and early August, it had gotten worse, and inhalers and breathing treatments weren't doing much. My PCP listened to my lungs and thought I had walking pneumonia and wanted to put me on antibiotics. I suggested an X-ray to be sure.

I was leaving after having the X-ray done when my doctor called me from her cell. The tech, upon seeing my X-ray notified the radiologist STAT for reading. I had a large plural effusion & partial collapsed lung. This wasn't registering with me that my cancer might have returned.

Then, my PCP said that she had called my oncologist, and he was expecting me. Say what??? I definitely was now having an oh-shit moment! How did we go from pneumonia to oncology involvement? She said she wasn't sure what was wrong, but since I was already established with oncology, he could get me seen by a pulmonologist quicker than she could because it was specialist to specialist.

I didn't have time to research anything at that point; I just needed to get to oncology. I called my boss to explain, as I was expecting to return to work after the X-ray, still not thinking about cancer or realizing the gravity of the situation.

I went to the oncologist. He wanted—and I needed—a STAT drainage of the lung, seeing that it was partially collapsed. The problem was, Interventional Radiology required a COVID test within 48 hours, or they wouldn't do a procedure. The only COVID tests being done were on inpatients, which complicated things.

I called my boss and let her know what was going on, and she told me to come back to work, and she'd test me. Oncology scheduled the drainage for the next afternoon, seeing I was going to get tested, but I was to bring the negative COVID test result back so he could include it with the order or they'd cancel it.

I went to work the morning of the drainage and left at lunchtime to go home so my husband could take me to have it done. Remember when I mentioned I have "strange reactions"? Well, partially through the drainage, I began to feel unwell. I started getting hot and nauseous, and just as I said, "I don't feel well," I passed out. It was a vasovagal reaction for some reason.

I also did a quick flatline to keep everyone on their toes. When I came to, I had IV access in my hand, a charge nurse taking notes, my APRN giving orders, and a crash cart next to me. They drained 1200 ml before I passed out, and they had to stop the procedure. They showed it to me; it looked like "normal fluid"—straw-colored, and I could see through it. By this point, I had researched pleural effusions and was pretty sure from all the causes it could be attributed to breast cancer stage 4.

I returned to work the day after the drainage, continuing my life as I knew it at that moment. Three days later, pathology confirmed what I had suspected, but my appointment was still a couple of days away to confirm what I was reading in "my chart." I was numb; in denial of what this stage 4 diagnosis meant to me, my life, and how things were going to change.

I went to my doctor appointment, alone, as my husband wasn't allowed up and had to stay in the parking lot. I was told officially that my cancer was back. Stage 4; treatable, not curable, and with a pleural effusion, my prognosis was poor. They did not give me a timeline. We decided on a port, chemotherapy, and scans of all sorts to determine where else the cancer was. He explained that a pleural effusion is usually the last place it goes, so he was expecting it elsewhere. I said no—I'm weird, and it's not anywhere else. He said, "That will be rare." Yep, that's me!!

As I left the office and was in the lobby, I called my boss. I needed to go out on FMLA. As soon as I said the words "my cancer is back, stage 4," I lost it. I was crying, and she couldn't understand most of what I was saying, but she knew something was wrong because of my emotional state. I sat in the lobby for a few minutes to collect myself and my courage, as I now had to go face the love of my life and tell him I have cancer again.

Unlike last time, treatments wouldn't stop with stage 4. I think he could tell by the way I was walking, as he met me outside the truck and just held me as we both cried. After we pulled ourselves together, I told him about the appointments I would need to make and had to go into work to download the FMLA papers. He just looked at me, as if I'd lost my mind—thinking I was worried about work right after being told I had stage 4 cancer. Yes! I was determined that this was merely a blip in my life, and I would return to work after chemo.

Then I had the hardest calls to make! My three daughters were all going to be told over the phone, as they were in three different states. I downplayed it the best I could not only for them but because I was still in denial of what this meant for my life.

I had all the scans, and as I thought, cancer was in the pleural fluid of my left lung only. I had an echocardiogram to clear me for chemotherapy.

The chemotherapy was AC, also known as the Red Devil. They placed the port, and I ended up getting the same APRN to do my port who had done my drainage. He asked if I was "ready to behave" and then asked me if it was okay if he explained to the team why he said that, as they had a confused look on their faces. The port was placed with local anesthetic and there were no issues.

It was done in the morning, and I went back to work afterward. I didn't want my FMLA to begin until the day chemo started, which was still waiting on insurance approval. While waiting for chemo approval, I made an appointment with an attorney to go over our trust and will from California to ensure they met all of Florida's requirements. It needed a couple of changes, but not a complete overhaul.

That was surreal to do, now that I was stage 4. It was more emotionally taxing than I had anticipated. At times, I'm not sure what I thought it would be. Chemotherapy began, and it wasn't as bad as I thought it would be. I kept myself medicated with anti-nausea meds 24/7, and thank God they worked. I was fatigued and constipated but not vomiting—winning!

My head began to feel tender after the first dose, so I cut my hair as close to my scalp as I could. Within the next 48 hours or so, all of my hair fell out, and the tenderness was gone. My counts dropped as expected, but they never dropped low enough to halt treatment. Everything changed about two weeks after my third infusion. I couldn't put my finger on it, but something was "off." I didn't feel right, but I chalked it up to the counts dropping and the chemotherapy side effects, which tend to worsen with each infusion.

The night before I was about to have my fourth and final infusion, I woke up to use the restroom in the middle of the night and felt queasy, so I went to the kitchen to get a Zofran. I felt like I was going to pass out, but I made it to the couch, and out I went. I thought I screamed for my husband before I lost consciousness, but I guess not, as when I came to, it was now dawn, and I could see it wasn't pitch-black outside. I have no idea how long I was out, nor do I know what time I got up.

When I came to, I was freezing—my teeth were chattering uncontrollably. I pulled two winter blankets off the back of the couch, curled up in a ball, and put a throw pillow in my mouth, as I was scared I was going to break my teeth with how much I was shivering. I tried yelling for my husband, but I was quaking so badly that I couldn't talk. I prayed not to die, as I knew I was bad but was unable to help myself. I thought, "As cold as I am, I must be going into shock." I either passed out again or fell asleep.

Our dog woke my husband up, and when I woke back up, I wasn't shivering anymore. I was still cold, but not hypothermically cold. I said, "ER now." He helped me into the truck, as I was weak, and I called my oncologist to let them know what was going on and that we had a 45- to 60-minute drive to the hospital or his office. I wanted to know if it was okay to self-transport or if they needed to call 911.

I was cleared for self-transport, and my husband broke speed laws, stopping for red lights, but once traffic cleared, we went through them and got there in about 30 minutes. I had a STAT echocardiogram that showed a clot in my right atrium. I was admitted to the hospital, as they wanted to do a TEE (transesophageal echocardiogram) to determine if it was a clot or a tumor.

They couldn't tell on the echocardiogram, and although a tumor is very rare, they needed to be sure. For once, I wasn't the "rare" patient; it was a blood clot. Chemotherapy was halted, and I was placed on blood thinner, Eliquis. This was mid-October 2020.

They then started me on Ibrance in mid-November. I wasn't thrilled with the thought of taking that drug, and just like AC chemotherapy, my internal alarm bells were going off, but I ignored them and took it—not as directed, though. I took it every other day. After 8 pills, again on Thanksgiving Day, I was eating and tasted blood. My gums were randomly bleeding. I called the oncology after-hours line and was instructed to come to the clinic on Black Friday. No shopping for this girl!

I went to the clinic, and my platelets were low. They transfused me with 2 units. Over the course of the next two weeks, I needed several transfusions. The doctor wanted to lower my dose, but I'd already reported my severe reaction and sent copies of lab reports to my specialty pharmacy, which filed a class 4 reaction report with the FDA and the manufacturer. I wasn't allowed to have that drug, even at a lower dose. My white blood cell count had also dropped to 0.04 after taking just 8 pills! It took several days of daily Neupogen injections to stabilize my white blood cell count.

In December, a TEE was repeated, and the clot had dissolved, so I was taken off Eliquis. A CT with contrast showed stable disease, and I felt good; my counts had stopped dropping, and I returned to work. Happy 54th birthday to me! Seeing this was the age cancer had taken my parents, I was ecstatic to return to work and carry on with life. They put me on an aromatase inhibitor, but the joint pain was horrific, along with night sweats and mood swings.

We tried another one—similar effects. Beginning in June 2021, I began feeling the need to be drained again, a repeat of 2020. This time, the IR team accessed my port prior to starting the procedure, so when I coded, they were ready. Yep, it happened. I was drained in late July. I didn't code that time—woo-hoo! In late August, I was drained again, but this time I coded.

It was time to go out on FMLA as the draining was becoming too frequent, and the AIs weren't working. Mid-September 2021, I was at home when I suddenly went into severe bronchial spasms. I did a breathing treatment, but it offered very little help; nonetheless, it slowed it down.

I went to my PCP, who was only ten minutes away. She heard no breath sounds on my left side; however, my oxygen saturation was 98%. It made no sense—my right lung was compensating. She sent me to the ER, where a full X-ray showed a fully collapsed lung on the left side with severe pleural effusion.

The ER doctor was sweet and allowed the IR team to take me and place a chest tube since after the chest tube, I would need a permanent indwelling catheter, and it would be easier for me if they did it all at once. That was great, as the IR team gave me twilight sleep, while the ER just used local anesthesia for the chest tube. Upon placing the chest tube, they drained 1500 ml immediately, and it kept draining. The fluid was full of blood, definitely filled with cancer cells, and didn't look like before. I was admitted for four days. By the fifth day, I was draining 500 to 600 ml a day, so they put in a PlurX drain and sent me home.

The doctor told me then that I'd most likely not make it to Christmas 2021. That didn't resonate with me, so I didn't believe it at all, nor did I tell anyone. I went home on palliative/hospice. I continued draining myself, and the fluid started getting lighter in color and less frequent. I was in a wheelchair if I needed to go anywhere outside my home, as my lung was "trapped" and wasn't working. I couldn't walk more than 50 to 100 feet without assistance.

In December, I resigned my position. Also in December, I quit draining. A repeat CT scan showed "stable" disease when compared to the previous CT just before the chest tube. By January 2022, the PlurX drain was removed, and I started treatment again. This time the doctor wanted to try Taxol; I did one dose, but nope! I lost my hair after just one dose, and it brought back the neuropathy I had in 2010 that took several years to go away in my feet.

This would be a long-term treatment, so I refused it—quality over quantity.

CHAPTER 14

Next up was Faslodex in February 2022. No issues until April 2022. We weren't sure what was going on, but I thought I might be dying by how I felt, yet labs and scans couldn't find anything wrong.

It all started with heat exhaustion after I got a flat tire on an 85-degree day and help was 45 minutes out. The following day, I felt fine, so I flew out as planned to California to see my daughter, surprise a friend for her 55th birthday, and attend another friend's wedding. I overheated again my first night there. I stayed at my stepdad's house, and he turned the AC off at night. I was sleeping on the couch downstairs, and aside from the front door or garage door, there were no open windows.

I was so sick by morning. I left and went to my daughter's house to cool off, eat, and sleep to recover. That didn't happen; instead, I got worse. My daughter was scared I was going to die on her couch. The fourth night after work, I heard her yelling at her dad on the phone to do whatever he needed to come get me—fly, drive; she didn't care, just come get me. I was devastated emotionally, realizing that what was supposed to be a wonderful trip was hurting my daughter so much.

Her whole life, I had been heat intolerant, and she'd seen it before, but not this bad or prolonged. I cried as I drifted off to sleep, as her fear was real, and I was unable to "snap out of it" to reassure her I was going to be okay. The next morning, I had her take me to the ER. The nurse gave me one unit of IV fluid and had the IV running wide open before the doctor ever came by. While awaiting labs, she hung another. The doctor finally came by and said to me, "You have stage 4 cancer; why are you here? What do you expect me to do?"

I was speechless, to say the least, and angry at the same time. He then said, "Your labs are fine. I'm discharging you—go home and follow up with your oncologist." WOW! I don't know what happened to care in California, but I had already changed my flight for the next day, as I was waiting in the ER. One way or another, I was getting my butt on a plane to go home!

The two units of fluid I received helped a lot. I felt about 45 to 50% better. It didn't last long, but long enough to get home. When I got back to my daughter's house, I started reading my lab results. They were abnormal!! I doubt he looked at them. I was severely dehydrated according to points in my labs, and my glucose was elevated, and I'm NOT diabetic. I made it home and saw the doctor; I was given two more units of fluid. The next day, another two units were given. That's six units over four days. I was still not okay, but now my labs were normal and not showing dehydration.

However, I still had extreme fatigue (worse than when I was on chemotherapy), nausea, and my blood pressure kept dropping. I asked if it was the Faslodex since I was no longer dehydrated. The doctor assured me it wasn't. I could NOT find anything close to what I was experiencing regarding side effects anywhere. Yet again, my gut was screaming at me every time I went to get that shot. I had my shot three days prior to these episodes, and I thought it had started after overheating and being dehydrated. However, I was still feeling bad even though I was hydrated.

If I wasn't asleep, I was on the couch nodding off. When I needed to visit the doctor, I had to lie down, as sitting made me feel queasy and like I was going to pass out. This went on until August, when I had an allergic reaction to the shot. They gave me steroids to counteract the reaction, and I began slowly feeling better overall. Faslodex is a long-acting treatment, so I was on oral steroids for two weeks. I was starting to feel better.

I delayed the September shot because our middle daughter was being promoted to Chief in the Navy, and she wanted my husband and me to pin her. That meant I needed to be well enough to travel to Virginia Beach. I was able to go—still in a wheelchair, but at least I was upright and feeling okay. After the allergic reaction and resuming the shots, my oncologist pre-medicated me with steroids and other medications to prevent any allergic reactions.

It worked until November 2023, when I reacted again. The nurse didn't even get 3 ml injected before I experienced bronchial spasms.

In December 2023, my doctor increased the pre-medications to the max dose, and I was okay; no reaction. I just felt fatigue after the steroids wore off, but not the non-functional fatigue like previous experiences.

In January 2024, I received the same dosing as in January for the pre-medications; however, the nurse got 1.5 ml injected before I had bronchial spasms. I required steroids and breathing treatments at home for close to two weeks before the breathing issues cleared up.

By February 2024, we went back to the aromatase inhibitors. It's hell, and based on my experience in 2021, I had no confidence it would work. Here we are in November 2024, and I was right—the PET scan shows progression for the first time since the December 2021 scan. It has spread to my liver, and I have a small pleural effusion. I feel fine; I have no symptoms of liver metastasis, but the biopsy confirmed it. I'm waiting for further testing on the tissue sample to see if it has any mutations that targeted treatments might work on.

I'm hoping so, as I am almost out of options, and the two options I know I have left are Verzenio and Kisqali. Ibrance was generation one, and these two are generation two and three in the same class. They have the same side effects as Ibrance, but based on my reaction to Ibrance, I'm hoping for a different outcome.

Chemotherapy is off the table due to my own blood clot history, in addition to family history. The doctor mentioned Taxol as an option, but not with the neuropathy that crept back after just one dose. That lasted almost five months.

Quality of life over quantity of life. My story isn't over yet, but I don't want to suffer just to add time, only for my family to suffer by watching me suffer because it's not quality time. I watched my mom go through hell for 362 days, rarely leaving the hospital while fighting AML. It almost destroyed me. Did it make me stronger? I'm not sure. I just know this isn't what I want to put my family through.

MEET THE AUTHORS

Marcella Powell

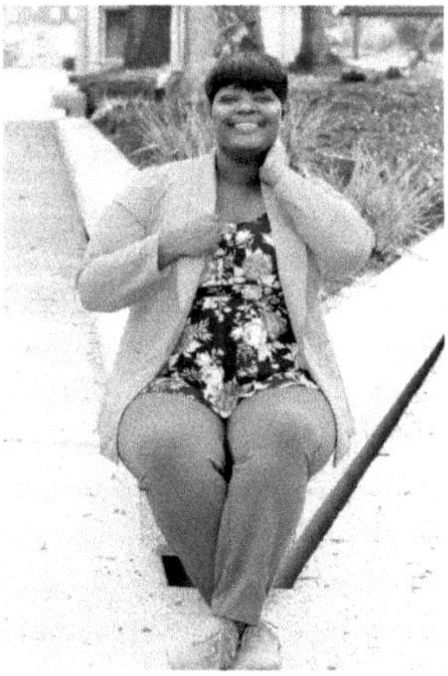

Marcella Powell is a native of Pensacola, Florida, and a two-time author. She currently serves as the President of Roar Performing Arts. Diagnosed at the age of 31 with HER2-positive, ER/PR-negative breast cancer, Marcella is now a proud survivor. She serves as a state leader for a national breast cancer foundation, advocating for research and awareness in the fight against breast cancer. In addition to her advocacy work, Marcella is a licensed minister, a mother, and a public speaker, sharing her message with the world that God is a God of miracles, signs, and wonders.

Fight Song: Love Me Wholly by Bishop S.Y. Younger

Tara Kamm

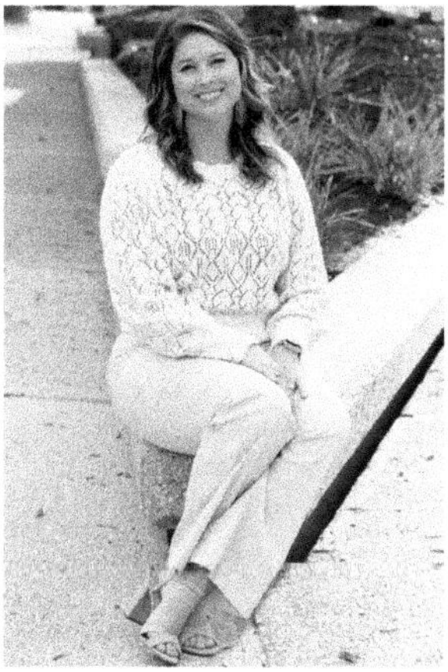

Tara Kamm has been a resident of the Gulf Breeze, Florida, area for the past 22 years, but she is originally from Huntsville, Alabama. At the age of 41, Tara was diagnosed with invasive ductal carcinoma breast cancer. She is the wife of Johnny, and together they recently celebrated 25 years of marriage. They have a beautiful family, with her son Joshua turning 20 this year and her daughter Kaitlyn turning 18. As they navigate this new season of having adult children, they love to travel and experience new things together as a family—always an adventure!

Tara has worked as a dental hygienist for the past 21 years and enjoys educating her patients on the importance of oral hygiene and its impact on overall health. She believes that the mouth is the window to the health of the entire body. In addition to her work in dental hygiene, Tara loves to explore new activities, especially in arts and crafts. There isn't anything she hasn't tried to make or recreate, as she views creativity as an essential outlet in her life.

Of all the things that define Tara, she hopes people will remember her for her love of Jesus and her desire to live a life that points to Him. Following her cancer diagnosis, she felt compelled to help others navigate the challenging world of breast cancer, which led her to start a YouTube channel and podcast called "Power Over Pink." In this platform, she interviews survivors to amplify their voices and provide hope and encouragement to others who may be facing a similar journey. Her fight song and morning alarm is a song by Hannah Kerr called "Warrior," which has served as a powerful reminder that she is unstoppable and a warrior.

Emily Hardin

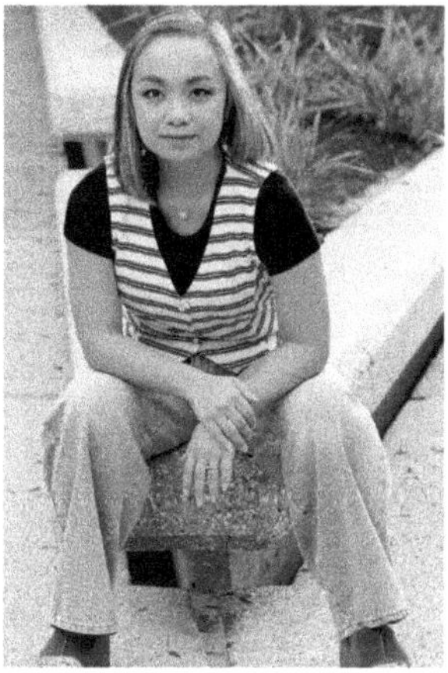

Emily Hardin was born in the Philippines and raised in Pensacola Florida since the age of four years old. Diagnosed with stage II Invasive Ductal Carcinoma in 2021, her breast cancer battle led her to open a store dedicated to cancer patients called The Boobie Boutique LLC.

She is a mother of two children, Rose and Raiden, and she serves as a Pensacola Breast Cancer Association Ambassador. Her hobbies include swimming at the beach, jogging with her dog, reading fiction novels and dancing around the house. She's most grateful for her ever growing relationship with God, her friends and family, and her mission to help empower women facing the many challenges of fighting breast cancer.

Fight Song: Brave by Hanna Ferm

Tina Piser

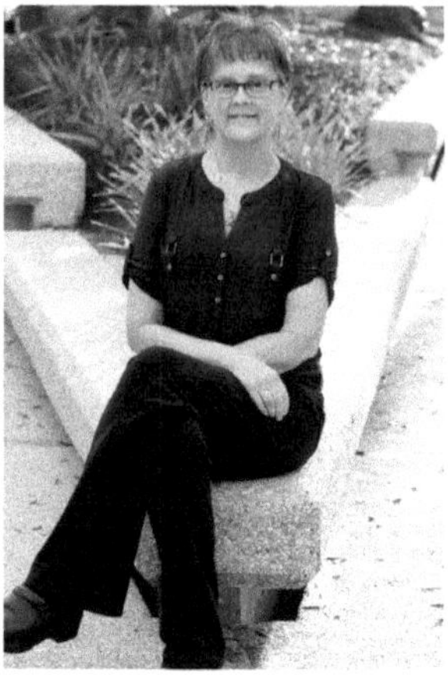

Tina Piser grew up in Orange County, California. At the young age of 21, she married a wonderful man and became a mother to two bonus daughters. Five years later, she welcomed her third daughter into the world.

Throughout her adult life, Tina has been a devoted wife and mother, a caretaker, and an advocate for her mother as she battled acute myeloid leukemia (AML). Tina also owned a pizzeria for ten years and worked as a phlebotomist and medical assistant for many years.

At 41, Tina received her first breast cancer diagnosis. At 50, she moved to Northwest Florida, and 3.5 years later, she faced a stage 4 breast cancer diagnosis.

In her spare time, Tina enjoys baking, meal prep cooking, canning, sitting outside to listen to the heavy rain, and taking quiet walks on the beach at night after it cools down.

www.ingramcontent.com/pod-product-compliance
Lightning Source LLC
LaVergne TN
LVHW050922210926
848482LV00012B/493
9798349349775